Challenges for Midwives

volume one

Also available in the 'Current Issues in Midwifery' series:

Psychology for Midwives by Ruth Paradice

Health-related Fitness during Pregnancy by Sylvia Baddeley

Obstetric Litigation from A–Z by Andrew Symon

Demystifying Qualitative Research in Pregnancy and Childbirth edited by Tina Lavender, Grace Edwards and Zarko Alfirevic

Perineal Care: An international issue edited by Christine Henderson and Debra Bick

HIV and Midwifery Practice by Jane Bott

Birthing Positions by Regina Coppen

Series editor: Jane Bott

Challenges for Midwives
volume one

edited by
Yana Richens

Quay Books
MA Healthcare Limited

Quay Books Division, MA Healthcare Limited, Jesses Farm, Snow Hill, Dinton, Salisbury,
Wiltshire SP3 5HN

British Library Cataloguing-in-Publication Data
A catalogue record is available for this book

© MA Healthcare Limited 2005
ISBN 1 85642 281 X

Printed in the UK by Biddles Limited, King's Lynn, Norfolk

Contents

List of contributors

Grace Edwards PhD, MEd Cert. Ed, ADM, RM, RGN is a Consultant Midwife at Liverpool Women's Hospital NHS Trust and Liverpool and Sefton Public Health Network and Principal Lecturer in Midwifery Research at the University of Central Lancashire. Grace.Edwards@lwh-tr.nwest.nhs.uk

Christine Henderson RM, RN, MA (Warwick), MTD, DPHE (Surrey), DipN (Lond) is Research Fellow at the School of Health Sciences, University of Birmingham, and editor of the *British Journal of Midwifery*.

Anne O'Donoghue BSc, RM, Cert Ed is a Registered Midwife at University Hospitals Coventry and Warwickshire NHS Trust. She is also the Service Co-ordinator for Pals in Pregnancy, a service for vulnerable pregnant women run by Coventry Teaching Primary Care Trust. ann.o'donoghue@coventrypct.nhs.uk

Rachel Rowe BA Hons is a Researcher at the National Perinatal Epidemiology Unit, University of Oxford. rachel.rowe@perinat.ox.ac.uk

Jenny McLeish is a Barrister-at-Law. She is Social Policy Officer at Maternity Alliance, 2–6 Northburgh Street, London EC1V OAY. Available online at: http://www.maternityalliance.org.uk

Anna Daley RM, DipHE, BSc is a part-time Staff Midwife at the John Radcliffe Hospital, Oxford.

Viv Gray RM, Dip HE Advanced is a practicing Midwife at the Whittington Hospital, North London. She co-founded and is a trustee of Birth Companions, a charity providing support to pregnant prisoners. viv@vivrosjas.fsnet.co.uk

Jane Morgan MA, ADM, Cert Ed, RM, RGN is a Senior Lecturer Midwifery and Research, Edge Hill College. morganj@edgehill.ac.uk

Janet Hirst PhD, MSc, PGCLTHE, RM, RGN is Lecturer at the School of Healthcare, University of Leeds. j.hirst@leeds.ac.uk

Jenny Hewison PhD, MA, BSc is Professor of Healthcare Psychology, School of Medicine, University of Leeds.

Yana Richens MSc, BSc, RM, RGN, SEN is Consultant Midwife in Public Health and Postnatal Care, University College London Hospital NHS Trust. yana.richens@uclh.org

Foreword

Further development in the public health dimensions of care is at the heart of the Maternity Standards of the National Service Framework for Children, Young People and Maternity Services (NSF), published by the Government in September 2004. In particular, those dimensions which relate to health improvement, reducing social and cultural disadvantage and tackling inequalities in access to and exclusion from, the benefits of good quality, appropriate, maternity care. The maternity standards within the NSF set the foundation for what must be common, high quality care across all maternity services. It has been widely recognised that over the last decade, midwives have been key and instrumental in developing needs led maternity services, focusing on women as individuals and tackling those issues which improve the social, health and mental welfare of women accessing care. If all services were at the level of the best, with strategies for addressing locally relevant public health challenges, then we would have a first class service. But there is some way to go to reach that goal across England.

There is much evidence that, effectively, addressing public health dimensions in care, before, during and in the months following birth, profoundly influences the health, well being and potential of children and the welfare of their families. The NSF offers midwives the opportunity to take up the challenge, to be at the leading edge of developments in public health aspects of maternity care and to develop strategically the quality and level of all services across England to that of the best.

It is clear in the NSF and in the Health and Social Care Standards and Planning Framework, that the Government expects new horizons to be set at local level, with local innovation and creativity encouraged and supported. It is anticipated that development of real choices for women, a focus on identifying and meeting relevant user needs and effective information exchange, will be at the heart of local improvement. It is expected that partnership working within and across services, will positively influence developments and that, what Government refers to as 'old institutional barriers' will not be allowed to stand in the way of creatively tackling the public health agenda which lies at the heart of the problems facing the NHS.

Midwives, at all levels and in all roles, need to be politically aware. Awareness informs our vision and increases opportunity to develop further cost effective services, focused on public health needs and on pregnancy as a normal life event, where unnecessary, costly interventions are reduced. Services which women want to use and which given them appropriate information and real choices, and that aim to meet their individual needs through pregnancy and childbirth and support them in their parenting role after birth.

This book has been written by experts, based on working knowledge from their own sphere of practice. It can act as a reference for midwives and for others contributing to the development of new dimensions in public health aspects of maternity care. It describes good practices which exist, and I am sure, it can assist those developing maternity services in their own localities. In particular, where these are focused on tackling the public health challenges which make a real difference for women, for children and for the health and welfare of their families.

Meryl Thomas
Co-chair, Maternity External Working Group of the National Service
Framework for Children, Young People and Maternity Services
Honorary Vice-president, Royal College of Midwives
November, 2004

Introduction

The key message of this book is that each and every pregnant woman wants safe, high quality care regardless of ethnicity, background, physical disabilities or cultural needs. The provision of safe, high quality care is the challenge for midwifery if we are to see a reduction in maternal mortality rates — recently highlighted in the Confidential Enquiry (Confidential Enquiry into Maternal and Child Health [CEMACH], 2004). This report provides stark evidence of the inherent inequalities in current maternity care provision. It confirms that women most at risk are those that are socially disadvantaged, excluded or vulnerable. Such women were the focus for this book.

Midwives are in a unique position because they deliver services across primary, secondary, tertiary and independent sectors. Because of the diverse nature of midwifery care, and the settings in which such care is delivered, midwives come into contact with women from many different ethnic and cultural backgrounds. As midwives we provide an important first contact for women.

This book is designed to help midwives care for women who are socially disadvantaged, excluded or vulnerable. Women who have been identified as being most at risk from maternal death include asylum seekers and women who experience domestic violence. These women need both our technical and our non-technical help, and we need to learn how to really listen to them and hear their stories. As midwives we must look beyond labels and stereotypes — only then will we begin to realise that we can truly make a difference to women's experience of pregnancy and childbirth.

Yana Richens
Consultant Midwife in Public Health and Postnatal Care
University College London Hospital NHS Trust
Elizabeth Garret Anderson and Obstetric Hospital
Huntley Street
November 2004

Reference

Confidential Enquiry into Maternal and Child Health (2004) *Why mothers die — 2000–2002*. CEMACH, London

Acknowledgements

I thank the wonderful contributors of this book, Binkie at MA Healthcare Limited for her enthusiasm and support. My dear friend Lynne who is always a sounding board. My husband Mark and children Megan, Jackson and Sam who make me happy to be a wife and mother, my father Mohammad and sister Marion whose memories only bring warmth and comfort.

1

Challenges facing midwives around public health

Grace Edwards

Introduction

There are many challenges that face midwives in their daily practice, but the challenge of working in a public health way is perhaps one of the most exciting and yet frustrating challenges. Successful implementation of midwifery public health practice requires patience (change doesn't happen overnight), working in partnership with women and their families in a truly empowered way and working in collaboration with other agencies and professionals.

What is public health?

First of all it is helpful to define what we mean by public health. In 1988, Donald Acheson described public health as:

> *... the science and art of preventing disease, prolonging life and promoting health through the organised efforts of society. Its chief responsibilities are the surveillance of the health of a population, the identification of its health needs, the fostering of policies which promote health, and the evaluation of health services.*

A more succinct definition is described by Derek Wanless as:

> *The science and art of preventing disease, prolonging life and promoting health through the organised efforts of society.*
>
> (Wanless, 2004)

Public health in the United Kingdom

Midwives are the main providers of care to women throughout pregnancy, birth and the postnatal period and have a distinct contribution to make to improve health. It has been recognised that they are ideally placed to work with women and their families across the whole community, to improve health care and to contribute to the reduction of health inequalities (English National Board [ENB], 2001). Because of this, it is vital that midwives understand how their practice contributes to the overall health of the communities in which they work, but also to be part of the developing Public Health Agenda.

One of the most important publications in terms of reforms to the NHS culture was the Government's report *Shifting the Balance of Power* (DoH, 2001) which introduced a 'bottom up' philosophy, with the balance of power being moved towards front-line staff and local communities. This introduced widespread changes to the structure of the NHS, leading to the following major initiatives:

❖ Primary care trusts (PCTs) became the lead organisations in assessing, planning and securing all health services. Each PCT has in place a Director of Public Health.
❖ NHS trusts provide services in agreement with their local PCTs. There is an emphasis on clinical networks and team working. High performing trusts will have the opportunity to apply for foundation status, and receive greater autonomy.
❖ The Strategic Health Authorities (SHAs) replaced the ninety-five Health Authorities (HAs), but are not directly involved in service planning, but provide the overall support for NHS agencies.

The major issues for midwives in public health focus around inequalities, poverty and lifestyle. But, for the first time, midwives are able to lead on midwifery public health issues and develop services with support from the best available evidence and Government report. This means that midwives are able to be directly involved and influence local policies and services around midwifery. This leadership potential is further strengthened by the National Nursing and Midwifery Strategy published in 1999.

The leadership role of nurses and midwives within the NHS was clearly highlighted by the Government publication *Making a Difference* (DoH, 1999). This described the creation of consultant nursing and midwifery posts to provide clear clinical leadership. The Government acknowledged the importance of nurses and midwives in delivering high quality care and described how it intended to extend the roles of nurses, midwives and health visitors particularly around prescribing, nurse-led services and primary care initiatives. Midwives are mentioned as having the potential to expand their roles to include wider responsibilities for women's health.

The links between public health issues, such as deprivation, nutrition and lifestyle are not new. In 1980, Sir Douglas Black published his report that highlighted the gaps in health and life expectancy between the richest and poorest in our society (Department of Health and Social Services [DHSS], 1980). He showed that men died earlier than women, and that both sexes from the lower social classes died earlier from cancers, heart disease and accidents. In fact, he stated that the risk of death before retirement is two-and-a-half times as great in class V (unskilled manual workers and their wives), as it is in class I (professional men and their wives). Perinatal and stillbirth rates for social class V were double those of social class 1. Twenty-five years later, nothing has changed. The Acheson report in 1998 found that mortality and morbidity was directly related to social class and poverty (Acheson, 1998).

Although there is recognition that where you are born and the social circumstances in which you live will affect your life, some of the facts around child health within the UK are still shocking.

In the UK there is still a north/south divide, with people living in the south of the UK generally enjoying better health than those who live in the north. A child born in Liverpool or Manchester will live, on average, nine years less than a child born in Westminster or Chelsea.

Over one in three children in the UK live in poverty. A third of children in the UK live with at least one adult smoker, but among low-income families the figure is 57% and the infant mortality in social class V is 77% higher than in social class 1 (Department of Health, 2002). Also, babies born to families in disadvantaged groups are more likely to be smaller. Babies with fathers in social classes IV and V have a birth weight which is on average 130 grams lower than that of babies with fathers in social classes II and I. Reduced growth in the womb has been linked with increased mortality and morbidity in the first year of life, and throughout childhood (Barker, 1998). The Acheson report also found that children born and brought up in families with low levels of educational attainment, material disadvantage or in lower socio-economic groups are likely to experience worse health in later life (Acheson Report, 1998).

Many Government reports describe the crucial influence of early life on subsequent mental and physical health and that policies which reduce early adverse influences on health may result in multiple benefits, not only throughout the life course of that child but to the next generation (Acheson, 1998; Townsend and Davidson, 1988; Confidential Enquiry into Maternal and Child Health (CEMACH, 2004).

The present Labour government has shown a real commitment to public health and supported these initiatives financially. As a result, several major publications have shifted the emphasis towards public involvement and empowerment in the NHS.

Saving Lives, Our Healthier Nation (DoH, 1999) was the Government's White Paper issued in response to the Acheson Report. It had the explicit aim of addressing the widening gap in health outcomes between the richest and the poorest groups in our society. It highlighted four major areas to be tackled, cancer, coronary heart disease, suicide and accidents. Smoking was mentioned as the major cause of premature death. There was an emphasis on a modern and expert public health workforce.

The *NHS Plan* was launched in 2000 and described for the first time, the formulation of national inequalities targets and new ways of working towards these targets. It acknowledges that many healthcare issues start at home, with people taking responsibility for their own health. The inequalities between the richer and poorer socio-economic groups in the UK were highlighted with particular reference to smoking and teenage pregnancy. The national target was to reduce inequalities in health outcome by 10% as measured by infant mortality and life expectancy at birth between the 'routine and manual' groups and the population as a whole by the year 2010 (DoH, 2000).

The *Priorities and Planning Framework for the NHS 2003–2006* (DoH, 2000) made three specific targets that midwives could tackle, namely:

1   Reduce by 1% per year the proportion of women continuing to smoke throughout pregnancy, focusing especially on smokers from disadvantaged groups.
2   Increase breastfeeding initiation rates by 2% per year, focusing especially on women from disadvantaged groups.
3   Reduce the number of teenage pregnancies by 15% by 2004 and half the rate of conceptions among eighteen-year-olds.

The implications for these targets on midwifery practice will be discussed later in the chapter.

A further report in 2003 by the Department of Health (DoH, 2003) gave specific, local targets for improving maternity and child health and child development, targetting the vulnerable and hard to reach groups. The challenges included improving access to maternity services, especially early antenatal bookings and take-up rates for women who may be hard to reach, such as poor women, women from ethnic groups and teenagers. The report also emphasised the importance of increasing the take-up and duration of breastfeeding for new mothers, especially those in low-income groups and black and minority ethnic groups, using link workers and community mothers schemes.

So what can we as midwives do?

There are several challenges around public health that midwives can address and the following pages will give the reader some idea of how to tackle these challenges.

The medical model as a public health challenge

In 1970, the Peel report was published which recommended that all births should take place within hospital (DoH, 1970). This resulted in a marked reduction in the number of women giving birth at home and a centralisation of birth in hospital settings. Community midwifery provides mainly antenatal and postnatal care with little intrapartum care. As a result, care offered has become increasingly service-led to adapt to the hospital system. Most midwives now work a shift system which leads to fragmented care and reduces the possibility of continuity. Care by midwives is also increasingly concentrating on the physical needs, which may result in an over reliance on medical opinion and the medical model of care.

Western society uses a medical model which sees health as absence of disease and which reduces the body and the whole person to a collection of separate systems, organs, tissues and cells. It usually concentrates on dealing with symptoms and not the cause of the problem. The National Health Service in Britain is based around the activities of specialists who concentrate on curing particular diseases. This model is mainly hospital-based.

There is no doubt that this model has enabled diseases and disorders to be identified and treated in a scientific way and has saved lives. A good example of this is the identification and treatment of diseases such as smallpox, which was a major killer in the last century. The model does improve some outcomes, but does not address other causes of ill health, such as social and public health factors.

Since pregnancy is essentially a normal, physiological event, midwifery does not sit easily within a medical model of care. The medical model tends to blame people for their own failings, such as smoking, poor diet and lack of exercise. It tends to treat the symptoms rather than look at health education, prevention and the social causes and doesn't address the problems that may affect health in the first place, such as poor diet, pollution and poor housing (Baggott, 1998). The patterns of care evident today in maternity practice are often referred to as 'the medical model of care', influenced by those who believe that birth is only normal in retrospect (O'Driscoll and Meagher, 1980).

The social model of health

Another model of health is the holistic or social model of health, which looks at the person as a whole and at other factors which might affect health, eg. lifestyle and living conditions. A public health approach is a good example of this. This model looks at the health and healthcare needs of communities and causes of ill health as well as treatment. It looks at the whole person, not just an isolated medical event.

It also recognises the fact that illness may mean different things to different people. Illness and health cannot be treated individually but are seen in the social and economic settings that people are a part of. Another important aspect of this model is that it recognises that social and environmental factors make some groups of people more vulnerable to disease than others.

A criticism of this model is that there may be too much attention paid to the social effects on ill health without recognising the contributions that medicine has made to the improvement of health (Baggott, 1998).

Self-empowerment model of health

There is a third model, the self-empowerment model. This model is concerned with empowering people to recognise the factors which might affect their way of life and taking responsibility for their health. Self-empowerment comes from within. If achieved, it enables the person to have a sense of ownership over their body, emotions, attitudes, knowledge and abilities (Baggott, 1998).

Self-empowerment during pregnancy has the potential to enable a woman to make choices and influence the care she receives. She becomes an active participant rather than a passive recipient of care. Seeking self-empowerment is not an easy option for women because ownership and responsibility are socially constructed concepts, which are used to define boundaries of behaviour. Consequently, for a self-empowerment model to succeed it needs the development of self-esteem and assertiveness within individuals and communities (Hall, 2003).

It is easy to suggest that midwives should adapt a social model on which to underpin their care but, in practice, this may not be that easy. However, Ball *et al* (2002) looked at reasons why midwives leave practice. Although the reasons were complex, the major reason cited for leaving was dissatisfaction with midwifery. Many midwives felt that they lacked control of their practice and could not practice autonomously. Working to a medical model of care will reduce control for midwives.

Midwives also need to value the diversity of each other's roles. If we do not support each other, we cannot effectively support the women in our care. If we work towards a social model of care, we put the woman and her family at the centre of care, not the service needs. If we work flexibly around the needs of the woman, we can have longer time at home. Many innovative units now practice annualised hours so that flexibility is possible.

One barrier to working in this way is fear. We are all fearful of change, even good change, but a cultural and philosophical change in midwives is needed to utilise our skills most effectively. We are practitioners of normal birth and normal birth doesn't tend to work around shifts!

Vulnerable women as a public health challenge

As previously mentioned, women from deprived or vulnerable groups are at a greater risk of mortality and morbidity during pregnancy and childbirth. The West Midlands has the worst deprivation in the country and also the highest number of people from ethnic minorities. In 1999, the combined death rate for babies was 11.5 per thousand total births, which is much higher than the more affluent area of Oxford which had a mortality rate of 9.6 per thousand births. The national average is eleven deaths per thousand births (Office of National Statistics, 1999).

National reports highlight some of the inequalities in health outcomes in childbirth. The Confidential Enquiry into Maternal Deaths (CEMD) (Confidential Enquiry into Maternal and Child Health [CEMACH], 2004) has once again shown that the poorest women in our society are more likely to die from childbirth. Women living in the most deprived areas having a 45% higher death rate compared to women in more affluent parts of the country. The report highlights that women from an ethnic minority are on average three times more likely to die, and that newly arrived refugees and asylum seekers have a mortality rate seven times higher than White women. In addition, 14% of deaths were from women who had declared that they had suffered domestic violence.

There was also an increase in deaths in young women under eighteen and a disproportionate number of deaths from traditional travellers. In addition, 12% of deaths were from women who had declared that they had suffered from domestic violence. The Confidential Enquiry into Stillbirths and Deaths in Infancy (CESDI) has shown that cot death is five times more likely if both parents smoke, that perinatal mortality is directly related to social class and that deaths in social class V are twice as high as in social class I (Fleming *et al*, 2000).

To care for women from vulnerable groups, an appreciation of the wider effects of health is need. A good way of appreciating these effects is by examining the wider determinants of health as described by Dahgren and Whitehead (1991). The wider determinants of health recognise the effects of outside factors on an individual's health. These include age, sex and genetic makeup. Personal behaviour such as alcohol use, smoking and exercise are also considerations. The effects of friends, relatives and the community within which they live can also affect the health of an individual, both negatively and positively. Wider influences on health include access to services, food supplies, living and working conditions. Finally, there are the cultural, economic and environmental conditions prevalent in society. All of theses factors interact with each other and have important influences on the health of the individual. An example of this is if a young woman becomes pregnant and smokes, she is unlikely to stop if smoking is the norm within her peer and family group. If a woman gives birth within a bottle feeding culture, she is unlikely to breast feed her baby.

Exciting initiatives such as 'Sure Start' are helping to address some of these determinants. Sure Start was set up as part of the national drive addressing inequalities to provide extra services to families in the 20% most deprived wards in the UK. It represents the first efforts in bringing together early education, childcare, health and family support for the benefit of young children living in disadvantaged areas and their parents.

The aims of Sure Start are:

* increasing the availability of childcare for all children
* improving health and emotional development for young children
* supporting parents as parents and in their aspirations towards employment (www.surestart.gov.uk).

Sure start is paving the way for children's centres which will build on existing good practice. A significant number of families with young children already benefit from good quality integrated services. Children's centres enhance these services and extend the benefits to more families — bringing an integrated approach to service delivery to areas where it is most needed (Department for Education and Skills [DfES], 2003).

One of the major drivers of Sure Start and the children's centre is empowering women and their families. This is something that midwives can help with: enabling women to engage in parenting positively. Midwives need to work closely with Sure Start programmes and other local strategies to ensure that midwifery care forms part of the multi-agency approach to family-centred care.

Smoking as a public health challenge

Addressing the issues around smoking in pregnancy is one of the biggest challenges midwives may have to tackle, particularly midwives who work in deprived areas. There is a clear correlation between social class and smoking. In social class I only 14% of women and 15% of men smoke. This rises to 33% of women and 45% of men in social class V. Fifty-five percent of lone mothers on income support smoke with the figure rising to 82% for women in prison. Homeless women, who are particularly vulnerable, have the highest rate at 90% (Bridgewood *et al*, 2000). This higher rate in smoking is matched by much higher rates of disease such as cancer and heart diseases (Smoking Kills; DoH, 1998).

The effects of smoking in pregnancy are well documented. There is evidence that smoking can increase the risk of ectopic pregnancy and risk of miscarriage by as much as 25% (Royal College of Physicians, 1992). In addition, some research suggests that there is increased risk of fetal anomaly and a rise in the incidence of placenta praevia (Williams *et al*, 1991)

The Confidential Enquiry into Stillbirths and Deaths in Infancy (CESDI) found that babies born to women who smoke are most likely to be born into the lower social classes and are five times more likely to die of cot death than babies of women who don't smoke (Maternal and Child Health Research Consortium, 2000). There are also well-documented morbidity risks to children's health with an increase in the incidence of asthma in childhood, an increase in the number of hospital admissions for respiratory infections, as well as an increase in the risk of middle ear disease.

There is also evidence to show that children who breathe second-hand smoke at home are less likely to perform well at school (World Health Organization [WHO], 1999).

A systematic review by the British Medical Association (BMA) highlighted a connection between smoking and breastfeeding. Mothers who smoke are less likely to start breastfeeding their babies and, if they do, they breastfeed their babies for a shorter time. Mothers who smoke produce less milk, and milk that is of a poorer quality. Even if a woman does not smoke, but is exposed to second-hand smoke, there is evidence to suggest that they will breastfeed their babies for a shorter time (BMA, 2004).

The Government has set very ambitious targets of reducing the rate of smoking in pregnancy from 23% to 18% by the year 2005, and down to 15% by 2010 (DoH, 1998). It appears that smoking is decreasing in older age groups but this trend is reversed in young women and this is a world-wide phenomenon. The World Health Organization (WHO) estimate that the number of women smokers world wide will triple over the next generation and that over half of all children are exposed to second-hand smoke (WHO, 1999).

So, what can we as midwives do to address this?

One of the most important qualities that a midwife can possess is to be non-judgemental. Smoking is addictive and many women will already feel guilty about smoking, particularly if she has problems in pregnancy. Research has shown that interventions provided by specialists as part of antenatal care are effective in increasing smoking cessation rates among pregnant women (Health Develoment Agency [HDA], 2002). However, advice should not be left to smoking cessation specialists. Women often report that they were not given any advice. In a report by the Health Development Agency, only 38% of women reported receiving advice on smoking cessation (HDA, 2002). A further survey suggested that no women received advice or support to stop smoking (McCurry *et al,* 2002).

It has been shown that even brief interventions by professionals reduce smoking rates and, provided that advice is given sensitively, women welcome advice and support. Coleman (2004) recommends using the five 'A's' approach:

• ask about smoking at every opportunity
• assess smokers' interest in stopping
• advise against smoking
• assist smokers to stop

• arrange follow up.

To appreciate why some women do not stop smoking in pregnancy it is helpful to explore the cycle of change developed by Prochaska and DiClemants (1986). The first stage is a precontemplation stage where people are not seriously thinking about change. It is very difficult to persuade people to change their behaviour if they are in this stage. The second stage is contemplation, where individuals are seriously thinking about change. This is a helpful stage to give information about smoking cessation. The third stage is the preparation stage where individuals are ready to change. This is followed by the action stage where there is an attempt to change. If this stage is successful, then the maintenance stage is reached where change is achieved. Successful change is achieved by moving through the stages. However, we need to remember that relapse is normal. Most individuals relapse back into the precontemplation stage around three revolutions before they stayed at the final stage (Prochaska and DiClemants, 1986; Prochaska, 1994).

Midwives also have an important role to play as role models. As the largest group of maternity care professionals, midwives are in a unique position to influence our clients who smoke. We also have more contact with women than any other care provider. The International Code of Conduct on tobacco control say of health professionals:

> *They should act as role-models for their patients, by ceasing to smoke, and by ensuring their workplaces and public facilities are smoke and tobacco-free.*

> (WHO, 1999)

A midwife who smokes is not only in denial about personal risks, he or she is ignoring the influence this will have on women and families in their care. Additionally, perceptions of midwives as smokers may present a negative role model, giving implicit reinforcement that smoking is not dangerous. However, an ex-smoking health professional will serve as an advocate for tobacco control.

Breastfeeding as a public health challenge

There is no doubt that breastfeeding has major implications for the future health of the nation. The Government has recognised the importance of promotion of breastfeeding in helping to reduce infant mortality and morbidity, not simply in nutritional terms, but in many other ways, some perhaps, not as familiar to midwives as others. Most midwives will know that evidence shows that breastfeeding helps protect the infant from gastro-enteritis and respiratory infections (Kramer *et al* 2001; Howie *et al,* 1990). Less well known perhaps is the growing body of evidence that has shown that breastfeeding lowers the risk of otitis media (Duncan *et al,* 1993), and the incidence of urinary tract infection in babies (Marild *et al,* 1990).

It is also worth highlighting the long-term effects on the health of the woman. Women who breastfeed are less likely to develop ovarian cancer (Gwinn *et al,* 1990) and pre-menopausal breast cancer (Beral *et al,* 2002).

So why do women not breastfeed and, if they do, why do they give up so soon?

In some way Britain could be described as a bottle-feeding nation with artificial feeding being the cultural norm. The UK Infant Feeding 2000 survey (Hamlyn *et al,* 2002) showed that although 70% of women did initiate breastfeeding, after four weeks three out of four women were using artificial milk to completely feed their babies or to supplement breast milk. The rate of initiation of breastfeeding is linked very closely to social class, with the higher social classes being most likely to breastfeed. In some more deprived areas there is a complete lack of role models for breastfeeding and women and their families may never have observed a woman breastfeed her baby. This may be very important as some research suggests that since breastfeeding is a practical skill, women may gain more confidence in their own ability to breastfeed rather than from reading or talking about it (Hoddinott, 1999).

A major reason why women may stop breastfeeding is because of conflicting advice. Often midwives give conflicting advice with the best intentions, but this undermines a woman's confidence in both midwives and her own ability. If midwives and maternity units sign up to the United Nation's Children's Fund (UNICEF's) Baby Friendly Initiative (BFI), then there is a commitment to give the same advice to women (www.babyfriendly.org.uk).

The ten steps described by UNICEF, if adhered to, would help ensure that women were given consistent and non-conflicting advice. The ten steps for hospitals are:

1   Have a written breastfeeding policy that is routinely communicated to all healthcare staff.
2   Train all healthcare staff in the skills necessary to implement the breastfeeding policy.
3   Inform all pregnant women about the benefits and management of breastfeeding.
4   Help mothers initiate breastfeeding soon after birth.
5   Show mothers how to breastfeed and how to maintain lactation, even if they are separated from their babies.
6   Give new-born infants no food or drink other than breast milk, unless medically indicated.

7 Practice rooming-in, allowing mothers and infants to remain together twenty-four hours a day.
8 Encourage breastfeeding on demand.
9 Give no artificial teats or dummies to breastfeeding infants.
10 Foster the establishment of breastfeeding support groups and refer mothers to them on discharge from the hospital or clinic.

There is also a seven-point plan devised by UNICEF that can be used as a basis for developing breastfeeding services in the community.

A crucial time for supporting breastfeeding women is around discharge home. Trained, community peer supporters who have themselves breastfed may be an invaluable source of support for women. These supporters would enhance the role of the midwife in supporting breastfeeding.

Midwives meeting the challenge

There is no doubt that midwives can make a valuable contribution to the public health agenda, whilst establishing the unique autonomy of our role. Below are some key statements to reflect upon. Consider how your practice relates to these aims:

❖ Ensuring that midwifery practice is closely aligned to the achievement of health improvement goals.
❖ Overcoming boundaries between professionals, organisations and communities to ensure effective service delivery focuses on health improvement.
❖ Developing multi-agency/multi-professional approaches to work through the achievement of common goals.
❖ Nurturing and sustaining partnerships to improve health.
❖ Developing local solutions to local issues by involving people and communities in decision making.
❖ Continually reflect and challenge practice to ensure best practice results in best outcomes for health improvement.
❖ Being vigilant about using the wider determinants of health models (Dahlgren and Whitehead, 1991), ie. adopting a social stance to health.
❖ Identifying those in most need and reducing inequalities.
❖ Increasing the flexibility of midwifery practice to ensure that practice responds to identified need (Edwards *et al*, 2004).

A modern public health function can only be delivered successfully by a multidisciplinary workforce that is focused on improving health and reducing inequalities in local neighbourhoods, and by working in partnership with local authorities and other agencies (DoH, 2001). This means midwives working as part of a team, not in professional isolation.

The good news is that midwifery public health practice and autonomy are supported by the National Service Framework for Children, Young People and Maternity Services (DfES, 2004). This reinforces a social model of care, where care is woman-centred and based on normality, based on a multi disciplinary partnership which is described as managed care networks.

Finally, questions we should reflect upon are summarised by delivering the best-midwives contribution to the NHS Plan (DoH, 2003):

❖ What does this women want/need from me today?
❖ Where is the evidence to underpin my decision and actions?
❖ How does what I'm doing fit with the services that other health & social care professionals are providing?

Midwives **are** public health practitioners.

References

Acheson D (1998) *Independent Enquiry into Inequalities in Health.* Available online at: http://www.official.documents.co.uk

United Nation's Children Fund (2004) *Baby Friendly Initiative.* UNICEF UK. Available online at: http://www.babyfriendly.org.uk

Baggott R (1998) *Health and Health Care in Britain.* 2nd edn. Macmillan Press Ltd, London

Ball L, Curtis P, Kirkham M (2002) *Why do midwives leave?* Women's Informed Childbearing and Health Research Group, University of Sheffield

Barker D (1998) *Mothers, Babies and Health in Later Life.* Churchill Livingstone, Edinburgh

Beral V (2002) Breast cancer and breast feeding collaborative reanalysis of individual data from epidemiological studies in 30 countries, including 50,302 women with breast cancer and 96,973 without the disease. *Lancet* **360**: 187–95

British Medical Association (2004) *Smoking and Reproductive Life. The impact of smoking on sexual, reproductive and child health.* British Medical Association, London

Bridgewood A, Lilly R, Thomas M, Bacon J, Sykes W, Morris S (2000) *Living in Britain: results from the 1998 General Household Survey. Office for National Statistics.* The Stationery Office, London

Coleman T (2004) ABC of smoking cessation Cessation interventions in routine health care. *Br Med J* **328**: March

Confidential Enquiry into Maternal and Child Health (2004) *Why mothers die — 2000–2002*. CEMACH, London

Dahgren G, Whitehead M (1991) *Policies and Strategies to Promote Equity in Health*. Institute for Future Studies, Stockholm

Department for Education and Skills (2003) *Children's Centres — Developing Integrated Services for Young Children and their Families Guidance*. DfES London

Department for Education and Skills (2004) *National Service Framework for Children, Young People and Maternity Services*. DfES London

Department of Health and Social Security (1980) *Inequalities of health. Report of a research working group*. DHSS London

Department of Health (1970) *The Peel Report*. HMSO, London

Department of Health (1998) *Smoking kills — A White Paper on Tobacco*. DoH, London

Department of Health (1999) *Saving Lives: Our Healthier Nation and Reducing Health Inequalities: an Action Report*. DoH, London

Department of Health (1999) *Making a Difference. Strengthening the role of nurses, midwives and health visitors*. DoH, London

Department of Health, (2000) *The NHS Plan: A plan for investment, a plan for reform*. DoH, London

Department of Health (2000) *The Priorities and Planning Framework for the NHS 2003-2006*. DoH, London

Department of Health (2001) *Shifting the Balance of Power: the next steps*. DoH, London

Department of Health (2002) *Improvement, expansion and reform — the next 3 years: priorities and planning framework 2003–2006*. DoH, London

Department of Health (2003) *Tackling Health Inequalities: A programme for action*. DoH, London

Department of Health (2003) *Delivering the best-midwives contribution to the NHS plan*. Department of Health Publications, London.

Department of Health and Social Services (1980) *The Black Report*. DHSS, London

Duncan B, Ey J, Holberg CJ (1993) Exclusive breast feeding for at least four months protects against otitis media. *Pediatrics* **91**: 867–72

Edwards G, Gordon U, Atherton J (2004) Developing the midwifery contribution to public health. *Br J Midwifery* (in press)

English National Board (2001) *Midwives in Action*. ENB, London

Fleming P, Blair P, Bacon C, Berry J (eds) (2000) *Sudden Unexpected Deaths in Infancy: The CESDI SUDI Studies 1993–1996*. The Stationery Office, London

Gwinn ML, Lee NC, Rhodes RH, Layde PM, Rubin GL (1990) Pregnancy, breast feeding and oral contraceptives and the risk of epithelial cancer. *J Clin Epidemiol* **43**: 559–68

Hall D (2003) *Health for all Children*. 4th edn. Oxford University Press, Oxford

Hamlyn B, Brooker S, Oleinkova K, Wands S (2002) *Infant feeding 2000. A survey conducted on behalf of the Department of Health, the Scottish Executive, the National Assembly of Wales and the Department of Health, Social Services and Public Safety in Northern Ireland.* Stationary Office, London

Health Development Agency (2004) *Smoking interventions for children and young people.* Taken from: Better health for children and young people. HDA briefing no 6, June 2004. HDA, London

Hoddinott P (1999) Why don't some women want to breast feed and how might we change their attitudes? A qualitative study (MPhil thesis). Department of General Practice, College of Medicine, University of Wales

Howie PW, Forsyth JS, Ogston SA, Clarke A, Florey CD (1990) Protective effect of breastfeeding against infection. *Br Med J* **300**:11–16

Kramer M, Chalmers B, Hodnett H, Sevovskas Z, Dzikovich I, Shapiro S *et al* (2001) Promotion of Breastfeeding Intervention Trial (PROBIT). *JAMA* **285**: 413–20

McCurry N, Thompson K, Parahoo K, O'Doherty E, Doherty AM (2002) Pregnant women's perceptions of the implementation of smoking cessation advice. *Health Educ J* **61**: 20–31

Marild S, Jodal U, Hanson LA (1990) Breast feeding and urinary tract infection. *Lancet* **336**: 942

Maternal and Child Health Research Consortium (2000) *Confidential Enquiry into Stillbirths and Deaths in Infancy (CESDI) 7th annual report.* MCHRC, London

Office of National Statistics (1999) *Trends in infant mortality in England.* ONS, London

O'Driscoll K, Meagher D (1980) *The Active Management of Labour.* Ballière Tindal, Eastbourne

Prochaska JO, DiClements C (1986) Towards a comprehensive model of change. In: Miller WR, Heather N, eds. *Treating Addictive Behaviours.* Plenum Press, New York

Prochaska JO (1994) Strong and weak principles for progressing from precontemplation to action on the basis of twelve problem behaviours. *Health Psychol* **13**: 46–51

Royal College of Physicians (1992) *Smoking and the Young.* Royal College of Physicians, London

Sure Start (2004) The Sure Start Unit. Available online at: http:// www.surestart.gov.uk

Townsend P, Davidson N (1988) *Inequalities in Health. The Black Report.* Penguin Groups, London

Wanless D (2004) *Securing good health for the whole population: Final report.* DoH, London

Williams MA, Mittendorf R, Lieberman E, Monson RR, Schoenbaum SC, Genest DR (1991) Cigarette smoking during pregnancy in relation to placenta previa. *Am J Obstet Gynaecol* **165**: 28–32

World Health Organization (1999) *International consultation on environmental tobacco smoke and child health: consultation report.* WHO/NCD/TFI/99.10. Available online at: http://www.who.int/topics/smoking/en/

2

The public health role of the midwife

Christine Henderson

Ask most midwives about their 'public health' activities and they will say that it is an integral part of their role. So integral that it is difficult to quantify. The extent of involvement in public health activities by midwives currently is variable and largely unknown. This chapter focuses on a study undertaken in the nineteen maternity units of the West Midlands between December 2000 and March 2001 that attempted to determine the baseline of public health role of the midwife (Henderson, 2001).

Study design and findings

There were two stages to the study. During the first stage focus groups were held with midwives to determine what they considered to be the public health role of midwives and what their thoughts were about the meaning of public health. Three focus groups were held with thirty-seven midwives who worked in hospital and community settings. From the work of the focus groups a questionnaire was designed to generate a mix of responses from heads of midwifery, community midwifery managers and midwives. A total of fifty-nine questionnaires were returned, a response rate of 61%.

It is clear from the findings that midwives, and particularly those working within the community setting, carry out an important public health function. Difficulties in separating out the public health role from other aspects of the role were evident in the responses by heads of midwifery, community managers and midwives. The type of involvement the midwife performed for each activity was divided into one of four discrete areas:

- health surveillance and problem identification
- counselling
- general advice about health and health promotion
- targeting populations and working with specific groups.

Each of these activities could be subdivided into four areas: support and screening, parent preparation, integrated working and involvement with specific groups. Midwives might be involved in one or more activities or areas depending upon their role and responsibilities (*Figure 2.1*).

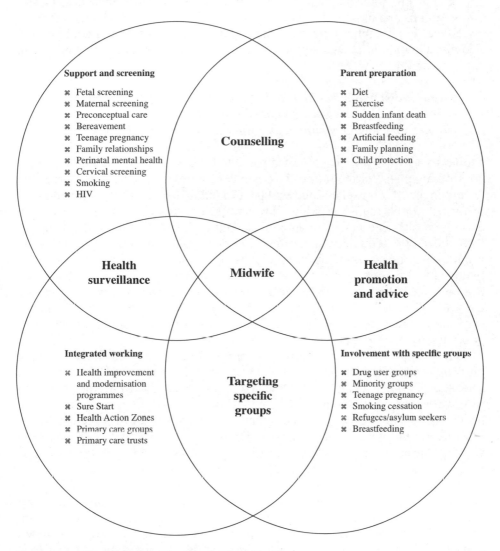

Figure 2.1: The public health role of the midwife

In the focus groups the consensus view was that public health i

and maintenance of health of an indivdual and their immedi

families. The promotion of healthy lifestyles has indirect

community generally and social circumstances, including hoi

were areas that midwives viewed as important to the promotion of health. Therefore, it was surprising that all midwives did not agree that health promotion was a public health activity. There was evidence that some midwives are providing specialist support to those particularly at risk of social exclusion and poor health, for example, teenage parents, travellers, drug abusers, minority ethnic groups and those living in poverty.

Eleven out of eighteen heads of midwifery stated that they did not have any midwives in their trust with a specialist public health role. The following quote summed up this view:

> *No specialist public health role but community midwives in*
> *particular undertake roles and advice which is part of what they do*
> *without specifically coming under the definition of public health.*

While some were looking to cater for needs of special groups others were considering plans for the future. Two heads of midwifery were considering the development of a consultant midwife post in public health. There were attempts to form 'action groups' working with health visitors and the plan to establish a public health lead in each community team and on hospital wards. A further three heads of midwifery stated that any plans were dependent on securing funding, or time and training for midwives. Three heads of midwifery indicated the need to reconfigure the maternity services and redistribute resources. They acknowledged the need for a radical restructuring of the way services are currently provided. Moving towards a multiprofessional approach, ie primary care centres, may be a way forward. There were concerns about fragmenting a good quality service that is provided currently.

There appears to be two forms of public health. An 'unofficial', largely unrecognised one, that midwives view as part and parcel of their existing role. On the other hand, there is the 'offically' recognised one that is linked to government priorities and funding. Commenting on increasing the public health role of midwives, community managers identified those which reflected local needs and government priorities. Domestic violence, extended postnatal visiting, breastfeeding, smoking cessation, parenting, and targeting vulnerable groups were all mentioned, including input into school curricula.

Initiatives where funding had been secured were clearly identified and the proportion of a midwife's time stated, for example, the Sure Start schemes. Eight units indicated that they were involved in health improvement and modernisation programmes and involvement in the schemes included participating in planning and input to bids. Thirteen units indicated that they had appointed midwives to schemes or that midwives had some input as part of a scheme. This included parent education, pre-school work, liaison with health visitors and breastfeeding. For some, Sure Start was a new and important area: at least five new schemes were being proposed where there would be midwife involvement.

Conclusion

The study endeavoured to establish a baseline of public health activities that midwives are involved in within the West Midlands region from the perspectives of heads of midwifery. community midwifery, managers and midwives. Part of the government agenda is to increase the public health role of the midwife. There is evidence that this is happening in places, sometimes on an ad hoc basis.

Although there are 'windows of opportunity' there are real issues to do with resourcing that need to be addressed. For some it is not a question of willingness, but one of being able to recruit and/or redirect resources in such a way that does not diminish the quality of services already provided. For others, it means a major upheaval for midwives to work in new ways. Respondents in the study indicated some of the areas where they would like to increase their public health role if given the opportunity.

The study highlighted the importance of adequate resourcing and the need to review the balance between midwivery and obstetric roles. Professional barriers need to be eliminated and there must be better collaboration and cooperation between professional groups and users. Midwives must be clear about their capability and capacity. Only by working as an integrated team with users will health inequalities be reduced, social exclusion be limited and public health become relevant and cost-effective.

Acknowledgement

This chapter is reproduced by kind permission of the *British Journal of Midwifery*.

Postscript

A further study was commissioned by the midwifery committee of the outgoing United Central Council and will be reported in *Challenges to Midwives, volume two* (Henderson, 2002).

References

Henderson C (2001) *The Public Health Role of the Midwife in the West Midlands.* Report presented to NHSE West Midlands, School of Health Sciences, University of Birmingham, Birmingham

Henderson C (2002) *The Midwifery contribution to public health in the United Kingdom.* Commissioned by the UKCC Midwifery committee. School of Health Sciences, Birmingham

Further reading

English National Board (2001) *Midwives in Action.* ENB, London

Royal College of Midwives (2001) The midwife's role in public health. Position paper 24. *RCM Midwives J* **4**(7): 222–3

Maternity Care Working Party (2001) *Modernising Maternity Care. A commissioning toolkit for primary care tursts in England.* Royal College of Midwives, Royal College of Obstetricians and Gynaecologists and National Childbirth Trust, London

Lavender T, Bennett N, Blundell J, Malpass L (2001) Midwives views on redefining midwifery 1: health promotion. *Br J Midwifery* **9**(11): 666–70

Bennett N, Blundell J, Malpass L, Lavender T (2001) Midwives views on redefining midwifery 2: public health. *Br J Midwifery* **9**(12): 743–6

3
Social support for pregnant women

Anne O'Donoghue

Introduction

This chapter will focus on the Pals in Pregnancy service, which provides social support for pregnant women living in disadvantaged circumstances. It will explore some of the issues around support for pregnant women particularly the ways in which peer supporters can help those who are disadvantaged and vulnerable, for example, teenage mothers, women experiencing domestic violence, those on benefits, asylum seekers and refugees. Pals in Pregnancy (Pals) is a new service offered by Coventry Teaching Primary Care Trust. This service is entirely different from the Patient Advocacy Liaison Service, also known as Pals. Pals in Pregnancy is co-ordinated by a midwife and employs local mothers to act as peer supporters. The service works in partnership with local midwives, health visitors and voluntary agencies.

Pregnancy is a time of change for a woman and her family. Women are faced with an array of choices from the moment they become pregnant; they have to decide on where to have their baby and whether to undergo screening tests. The number of decisions to be made can be bewildering for even the most assertive woman. Women, such as those on a low income, teenage mothers and women whose first language is not English may face so many other obstacles in their lives that they may not feel able to ask questions or they may be unaware of the different services that are available. In 1994 a consultation exercise was undertaken by Coventry Health Authority with the aim of improving access to the maternity services. It sought the views of local women and found that women wanted to talk to someone who understood their situation, was non-judgemental and would just be there for them (Schonveld and Kingswell, 1996). The Pals in Pregnancy service was developed to meet this need and has since been expanded to include other disadvantaged groups such as asylum seekers.

Social support

The concept of providing social support to pregnant women is not new and Oakley (1998) stated that providing support to pregnant women living in disadvantaged circumstances was beneficial to the health of the mother and baby. However, some women may regard the offer of support from professionals as intrusive and research shows that support given in this context may have a negative effect (Cohen and Wills, 1985). Professionals may offer support, which is not helpful, and in many cases interventions, although well intentioned, may be counter-productive (Oakley, 1992). Conversely, where support is perceived as being adequate it has been shown to equate positively with physical or mental health (Barrera, 1986; Hirsch and Rapkin, 1986). Abrams study (Bulmer, 1986) argued that public services should recognise that professionals are not the main source of social support and they should facilitate the formation of support networks consisting of family, friends and neighbours (Bulmer, 1986). Schumaker and Brownell (1984) define social support as:

> *An exchange of resources between at least two individuals perceived by the provider or recipient to be intended to enhance the well-being of the recipient.*

Pals offer information and emotional support to women to enhance their self-esteem. Initiatives such as New Deals for Communities, Sure Start and Children's Centres recognise that good social support can improve health (Department of Health [DoH], 2003).

Pals in Pregnancy

Pals in Pregnancy is targeted at women living in designated priority localities within the city; these include four 'Sure Start' areas and a 'New Deals for Communities' regeneration area. Within the priority neighbourhoods the rate of teenage pregnancies and low birth weight babies tends to be higher than average and there are more children aged 0–1 year in these areas. Priority neighbourhoods also have high infant mortality rates (Coventry Statistics, 2004).

The service is co-ordinated by a midwife whose role includes the recruitment, training and support of Pals, together with service promotion, audit and service development. Pals in Pregnancy is a flexible, non-judgemental and woman-centred service that offers different levels of support according to the needs of each client. Women can choose to have one-to-one support, telephone support or a combination of the two. Support is offered throughout pregnancy, for an hour a week or two hours every fortnight, and for up to three months after the birth of their baby. Evaluation of the service has highlighted that women who have used the service have found this particularly helpful, especially those having their first baby. One reason for this may be that midwifery care often ceases soon after the baby is ten days old, and before the mother has established a relationship with her health visitor. New mothers often feel isolated and vulnerable as they adjust to the demands of caring for a new baby and they value the support they get from their pal.

Referral to the service is by midwives, health visitors or voluntary agencies, such as those supporting asylum seekers or refugees. The service is offered to pregnant women who meet any of the criteria below:

- asylum seekers/refugees
- teenagers
- lone parents
- women living on benefits
- victims of domestic violence
- women whose first language is not English
- women who are homeless or living in a hostel
- women who have little social support
- professional discretion (eg. previous postnatal depression, stillbirth or low birth weight baby).

Ideally, women are referred at an early stage of pregnancy and the co-ordinator to assigns a pal to support the woman. Factors taken into account include social and cultural circumstances and whether English is the woman's first language. The pal and woman should speak the same language but interpreters are available when needed. Family members are never used as interpreters as this may inhibit a woman (Confidential Enquiry into Maternal and Child Health [CEMACH], 2004). Having received a referral the pal makes contact with the woman, usually by telephone, and discusses what type of support is required. The woman can change her mind about this at any time and it is common for a woman to start off with telephone support and then decide they want face-to-face support once they have established a relationship with the pal.

Pals usually give women their personal mobile telephone numbers so that they can contact them at any time if they have a problem. This is not usual practice within the health service and illustrates the commitment of the service to supporting disadvantaged pregnant women. None of the pals have ever received inappropriate calls from women and, for many, just the fact that they can contact someone in an emergency is enough to give them the confidence to deal with a problem. It can sometimes be difficult for women to talk freely at home, particularly if other family members are always present, so women may choose to meet their pal in a café or similar location. The service will meet the cost of refreshments due to the low income of many of the women using it. All the information exchanged between the pal and the woman is confidential, the only exception being anything that raises child protection concerns, which is made clear to the woman at the outset. The role of the pal does not include providing domestic help, baby-sitting or shopping. Sometimes it can be difficult for a pal to say no to help in this way, particularly when she has spent a lot of time with the woman. To help pals deal with this type of situation their training includes assertiveness skills and setting boundaries.

Recruitment and training

Pals are employed on flexible working contracts, enabling them to work at times that are convenient to themselves, their families and the women they are supporting. This way of working does have drawbacks in that it can be difficult to plan work effectively, for instance, matching clients with a pal especially during holiday periods.

The training for new pals is comprehensive and includes the working of the maternity services in Coventry, confidentiality, data protection, welfare benefits, personal safety, domestic violence and listening skills. Trainees are given the opportunity to practise their listening skills through enacting scenarios taken from practice and new pals are mentored by their more experienced colleagues when they begin visiting clients. Women are paid for the training and childcare costs can be reimbursed. The training takes place over six half-days and a final decision on suitability for the post is made at the end of the training period. This also allows the recruits time to decide whether the job meets their expectations. Pals attend monthly meetings where they receive support and ongoing training, which has included the benefits of breastfeeding, the effects of smoking in pregnancy and how to deal with stress. A session has also been included on baby massage to encourage women to interact with their babies since it has been suggested that this may be a beneficial intervention for those with postnatal depression (Onozawa *et al*, 2001). The service is keen to promote healthy lifestyle messages, but in a sensitive way that takes account of women's own priorities. Many of the women who use the service know about the effects of behaviours such as smoking in pregnancy, and some have admitted under-reporting how much they smoke to avoid the disapproval of health professionals. Therefore, it is important for pals to give information sensitively and only if requested by the woman.

Visiting policy

The Pals in Pregnancy service is flexible and designed to meet the needs of the pregnant women, this means that pals may visit at weekends or in the evening. To ensure their personal safety a detailed visiting policy has been developed. Initial referrals are received and scrutinised by the co-ordinator and if there are any identified risk factors, such as domestic violence, further information is sought before the client is allocated to a pal. If appropriate, the co-ordinator will accompany the pal on the initial visit and a risk assessment is undertaken, involving an appraisal of the area, the woman's living conditions and obtaining information on who else lives in the house. If there are no identified risks the pal arranges to visit the client. When the policy was initially developed the co-ordinator accompanied the pal on all primary visits. This proved to be time-consuming for the co-ordinator, intimidating for the woman and made it difficult for the pal to establish a relationship. It also meant that the pal could not arrange the first visit until the co-ordinator was available which made the service inflexible and caused delays. A review was undertaken and referral forms were redesigned to allow referring agencies to identify any known risks on the form. It was decided that accompanied primary visits would only be undertaken where there was an identified risk, such as someone with a history of violence living in the home or where the referral came from an unknown individual rather than a professional. Accompanied visits may still be undertaken where the pal or co-ordinator feel it is appropriate, for example, if the client wants an evening visit and the pal is unfamiliar with the area. Pals are not allowed to visit without letting the co-ordinator or another pal know where they are going and their expected time of return. For visits that take place outside of office hours, Pals in Pregnancy operates a responsible person system whereby each pal nominates a friend or family member who agrees to contact the co-ordinator, service manager or on-call duty manager if the pal does not return by an agreed time. The police would be contacted if the pal could not be reached within thirty minutes of the original check-in time. All the pals are conscious of their personal safety and adhere to the guidelines; there has never been an incident of a pal not returning from a visit as planned.

Service evaluation

A series of questionnaires have been developed in conjunction with the audit department to evaluate the service. There are pre- and post-service questionnaires which are used to collect information about the age of the client, ethnicity, living accommodation, health, alcohol and cigarette use plus the pregnancy. The questionnaires have been designed to be easy to use and consist mainly of multiple choice tick boxes. There are three post-service confidential questionnaires, the appropriate one is issued depending on the type of support received by the client (one-to-one, telephone or a combination of both). Obtaining completion of the pre-service questionnaire is straightforward since it is undertaken at the first visit. Completion of the final questionnaire has been problematic. There are many reasons for this, sometimes women move away without informing anyone or they terminate contact with their pal before a final meeting has been arranged. It has been particularly difficult to get the confidential questionnaire completed and returned. Initially, the confidential questionnaires were sent out by the co-ordinator with a reply paid envelope. However, the response rate was virtually zero. To overcome this problem the pals now issue the questionnaire at the penultimate visit and collect it at the final visit. The questionnaire is handed over in a sealed envelope to ensure that the client's answers are confidential. This has improved the return rate of the questionnaires and will enable the service to assimilate valuable information on which to build for the future. The data referred to in this chapter was gathered from May 2002 to August 2003, during which time 119 referrals were received and sixty-nine women accepted the service. The service was declined by the other forty women or they did not respond to the contacts made by the pal. The cost of the service during the sixteen-month period was £39,435 which equates to approximately £571 per client, taking into account only those who accepted the service.

Pals maintain confidential diaries in which they record details of their discussions with clients and any information that they have been given. The data are used as part of the service evaluation and women are told that the information they give is held securely. To ensure confidentiality, clients are identified only by their initials and all records are stored in accordance with the policies of the primary care trust. Pals submit monthly reports and hand in their diaries at the end of each year. These records are invaluable as they provide rich data which complements the information gathered by the questionnaires. Pals' diary entries show that women most frequently talked about their emotional state followed by their physical health, housing problems and requests for information or advice. The qualitative data collected shows that women valued the help and support they received from their pal. One woman stated:

My pal helped me to see the positive and I don't know what I would have done if I had not had a pal.

Mental health

About 13% of women experience postnatal depression (O'Hara and Swain, 1996) and although its duration is likely to be short (Cooper *et al*, 1991) it may have a damaging effect on the relationship of the mother and child (Murray *et al*, 1996). The antenatal period offers a unique opportunity to identify problems and initiate interventions aimed at ensuring secure attachment between mother and child. It has been argued that antenatal interventions are beneficial because pregnant women need support and display their emotions more readily and do not already feel that they have failed (Egeland and Erickson, 1990; Erickson *et al*, 1992; Egeland and Erickson, 1993). Not all interventions have been shown to be beneficial and routine screening to predict postnatal depression is not recommended (National Institute for Clinical Excellence, 2003). The Edinburgh Postnatal Depression Scale (EPDS) is used to screen emotional well-being (Cox *et al*, 1987), and is one possible tool to identify emotional disturbances (Holden, 1994) which has been validated for antenatal use (Murray and Cox, 1990). Murray and Cox (1990) suggest that women who score above fourteen antenatally and twelve postnatally are at increased risk of depression. Green and Murray (1994) expect 12% of women to be above threshold antenatally and 14% postnatally. In the pals group, 58% of women scored above the threshold antenatally and postnatally the figure was 50%. The high scores are not unexpected since the women referred to the service are disadvantaged and vulnerable. Encouragingly, the women demonstrated an improvement in their scores. This is contrary to the result expected and suggests that the service has a positive effect on mental health. This is supported by the post-service questionnaires in which 79% of women reported that they had a 'very good' relationship with their baby.

The advantages of the EPDS are that it was designed specifically to identify postnatal depression, it is usually understood by clients, it is short and it is widely used (Seeley, 2001). However, depression is perceived differently in other cultures and the application of the scale to women of different cultures has been questioned (Bashiri and Spielvogel, 1999). The EPDS has been translated into a number of languages and some ethnic distinctions have been noted, for example, O'Hara (1994) found that it was difficult for Icelandic women to identify the differences between some of the questions. There were also problems when the scale was used with Japanese women who are inclined to report medical rather than depressive symptoms when they are depressed (Yoshida *et al*, 1997). Bashiri and Spielvogel (1999) conclude that while the EPDS is a valuable tool for screening western women, care should be used when employing it with other cultural groups. Problems may arise with translation and conceptual equivalence when applying this to different cultures. The authors point out that the studies did not measure self-reporting symptoms. The EPDS does not consider these factors. They suggest that although the studies they examined did not measure whether women were comfortable with the self-reporting of symptoms, this could be a factor in the low sensitivity of the EPDS in non-Western women. Despite its weaknesses, the EPDS takes account of the changes caused by pregnancy, it is short and easily administered and is a useful tool for professionals to use so long as they are aware of its limitations.

Service users

The largest group of women referred to the service were asylum seekers and refugees (24%), followed by teenagers, young women aged thirteen to nineteen years inclusive (20%). Of the asylum seekers, 77% accepted the service while 58% of teenagers used the service. Pals in Pregnancy maintains links with local services that offer an educational course for young mothers at a local college. The service liaises with the refugee centre to assist pregnant asylum seekers and refugees.

Case study

I will now outline the circumstances of one client to give an insight into the work of Pals. Every woman is an individual and each one's circumstances are different so the case study I have outlined is unique. The names and specific features that could identify the client have been changed to ensure anonymity.

Hansa is an asylum seeker from the African continent whose first language is French, although she speaks some English. Hansa was referred to Pals in Pregnancy by her midwife and has been supported by Angela, one of the pals. On receiving the referral, Angela contacted Hansa by telephone and arranged to visit her the next day. Hansa was delighted to meet Angela and was very open about all her problems. She was tearful as she told Angela that she had been forced into a marriage and been physically abused by her husband. She had spent time in jail where she was sexually assaulted and she fled to the UK, leaving her child behind, to seek asylum. Hansa was relocated when she was five months pregnant, she knew no one, had many physical and emotional problems. She also had financial problems as her benefit money came through sporadically and at one point she had no money or food and her home had no hot water or heating. Hansa was boiling water and carrying it from the kitchen to the bathroom to try and bathe, obviously this was unsafe. The weather was cold so the lack of heating was a serious concern. Hansa had no idea how to contact her landlord or what to do when her benefit did not arrive. At the initial visit Angela ascertained who the landlord was and arranged for them to carry out essential repairs. The following week she accompanied Hansa to the refugee centre and helped her to make contact with the National Association for Asylum Seekers and Refugees. During her pregnancy Hansa had constant back pain and symphysis dysfunction made it difficult for her to walk far. About a month before the baby was due Hansa received a letter telling her to be ready to leave her accommodation in three days time as she was to be moved to a new location. There was no information as to her destination and she was distraught in case she was again moved to a new city. Angela supported her and helped her to find out that she was being relocated within the city. Angela liaised with the community mental health team and Hansa asked her doctor to refer her for counselling as a result of her discussions with Angela. Angela took Hansa shopping for baby items and showed her where she could obtain items that were reasonably priced. She also introduced her to the local church and Hansa received assistance from the parish visiting team. As a result of her referral to Pals in Pregnancy, Hansa was able to establish a network of support so that when her baby was born she was less isolated. She has had to travel to London periodically in connection with her asylum application which she has found stressful, particularly with a small baby, but this network has supported Hansa with her asylum application. She has become part of the local community and her English has improved. Throughout the time she was supported by Angela, she developed a relationship with her, contacting her whenever she had a problem. Hansa has absolute faith in Angela and knows that she can rely on her to help at any time. Although the future is uncertain, Hansa has been well supported throughout pregnancy and during the first crucial months of her baby's life. She has an excellent relationship with her baby and is much more positive about her ability to provide a stable environment for them both.

Domestic violence

The service has received referrals for women who have experienced domestic violence. Once women started to use the service and established a relationship with their pal they were able to disclose issues of abuse in their relationships. Domestic violence is a major public health issue and there is evidence that violence starts or increases in pregnancy (Bewley and Gibbs, 1998; Mooney, 2001). The Confidential Enquiry into Maternal Deaths 1997–1999 (CEMD) (RCOG, 2001) highlighted:

❖ Forty-five of the three hundred and seventy-eight women in the report had voluntarily reported violence to a healthcare professional during their pregnancy.

❖ None of the women who died had been routinely asked about domestic violence.

❖ Eight women were murdered by partners or close relatives, two others probably died as a result of medical conditions that arose because of domestic violence.

❖ Many women experiencing domestic violence booked late for antenatal care and attended appointments infrequently.

❖ 80% of those under the age of eighteen had suffered physical or sexual abuse in the home. All the girls under age sixteen had been abused by someone in the family.

Women who experience domestic abuse are more likely to suffer anxiety and depression (British Medical Association, 1998). They are also more likely to smoke, drink alcohol and use drugs in pregnancy. These behaviours may contribute to intrauterine growth restriction and premature birth (O'Donnell *et al*, 2000), and impact on the long-term health of children and women's ability to care for them. Pals are trained to be sensitive and make appropriate responses if a woman discloses domestic violence. They support women in a non-judgemental and non-directional manner while striving to empower them to make their own decisions. Information on local services available to women who are experiencing domestic violence is provided and pals are able to signpost women to other agencies. The flexible approach of the service is helpful because pals will visit or telephone women at a time that suits them, this may be when the partner is not present. Some service users just want to talk about their situation, although they are not ready to make the decision to leave. Pals are well informed about the availability of local services for women experiencing domestic abuse and they understand the importance of allowing women to reach their own decisions (Price, 2003).

The role of the pal can be stressful in these situations and it is important that they are well supported. Regular meetings with the co-ordinator provide them with the opportunity to debrief and discuss issues in depth. Pals are positively encouraged to contact the co-ordinator if they have any concerns. The job is rewarding and pals have stated that they get a great sense of achievement from seeing a woman they have supported take control of her life. Women that have used the pals service have entered further education, started to learn English and found employment as a result of information that their pal gave them. For the pal, too, there are many benefits. They become more confident and assertive, learn how the benefits system works and how to negotiate with different agencies in the city.

Inequalities in health

The work done by Pals in Pregnancy fits strategically into the Government's health improvement targets (CEMD, 2001; CEMACH, 2004; DfES, 2001), which include:

* Improve asylum seekers and refugees access to maternity services.
* Support vulnerable young mothers to develop healthy eating and nutrition skills.
* Increase the initiation of breastfeeding by 2% a year.
* Raise awareness of domestic violence, substance misuse and alcohol use in pregnancy.
* Achieve a 1% reduction of pregnant smokers year on year.
* Achieve a 10% reduction in smokers in 'Sure Start' areas by 2010.

Smoking and alcohol

Smoking is associated with a 30% increase in pre-term delivery; smoking and alcohol consumption are linked to social disadvantage plus a decrease in birth weight (Spencer, 2003). Nine women who used Pals in Pregnancy smoked but only two wanted help to give up and their names were passed to the smoking cessation midwife. The number of cigarettes smoked each day was quoted at between three and fifteen but all the women indicated that they had under-reported the number to their midwife because they felt guilty about smoking. They knew smoking was harmful but felt unable to cope without a cigarette. Although women have access to a specialist smoking cessation midwife, smoking is associated with social disadvantage and influenced by family and friends (Spencer, 2003). Consequently, it can be difficult for women to change their behaviour, particularly where smoking is the social norm among their peers. While only a couple of women disclosed alcohol use in pregnancy one woman did receive help from the Community Alcohol Service as a result of information received from her pal, and she was able to stop drinking alcohol in the pregnancy. More frequently, women were affected by a partner's alcohol consumption, this was a difficult issue for them to tackle especially as in many cases confronting a partner was likely to lead to domestic violence.

Infant feeding

The Infant Feeding Survey (DoH, 2000) confirmed the link between breastfeeding, a mother's age, educational level and social class. Mothers who left full-time education at the age of sixteen years and those in manual occupations (social classes 111 to V) were least likely to breastfeed. Pals support and encourage women to continue with breastfeeding, but while many women start breastfeeding they often do not continue. This is an important area where pals can help women who may be reluctant to approach professionals. They have had a talk from the infant feeding advisors from the local hospital trust and they are able to inform women about the benefits of breastfeeding and the specialist support available. Although the numbers of women using the service who breastfeed are low, it is encouraging to see that 61% of those who initiated breastfeeding were still breastfeeding their babies at three months. The service is investigating the possibility of training pals as peer breastfeeding supporters to enable them to develop their health promotion role and improve the long-term health of babies.

Nutrition

Many women, particularly asylum seekers, stated that they could not afford fruit and vegetables although most of them were aware of what constitutes a healthy diet. The questionnaires showed that:

- seven women ate no fruit and vegetables
- twelve ate one portion a day
- only four ate the recommended five portions a day.

Pals understand the importance of good nutrition and encourage women to eat fruit and vegetables and can signpost women to the community dieticians if they want information about how to cook and eat healthily on a low budget. In an effort to improve the diet of those on low incomes, Coventry is taking part in a scheme to subsidise fruit and vegetables and Pals will be instrumental in ensuring that the women they are supporting are included in the scheme.

Social circumstances

Of those using the service in 2002–2003:

- 53% of women using the service were not living with a partner
- 58% of women had been at their current address for less than a year
- 62% were living in rented accommodation
- 81% of women had no access to their own transport.

As so few women have access to their own transport they frequently have difficulty accessing parent education or attending clinic appointments. This contributes to social isolation particularly if women are new to the area, for example, asylum seekers who have no control over where they live. They frequently arrive in the city knowing nobody and with no idea of what services are available or where they can go for help. Pals in Pregnancy has been able to help women access services within the city and obtain items of baby clothing and equipment.

Women are encouraged to attend parent education classes and, on occasion, Pals have helped women attend. Many of the women using Pals in Pregnancy do not attend parent education, they often feel uncomfortable in groups where most of the others are couples (53% of women do not live with a partner and, if they do, often the partner is unsupportive). Pals can help by attending classes with women. This is important as it empowers women and gives them confidence in their ability to care for their babies. If a woman is well prepared for motherhood she may require less support from other professionals, such as midwives and health visitors, and if problems are identified early, appropriate strategies can be employed. Nationally, there is a shortage of midwives and so a service like Pals in Pregnancy can help by supporting women and easing the workload of midwives. Some may see this as an erosion of their role but many will acknowledge that such a service is beneficial to women. This is because the service has a wide remit, it is flexible and woman-led, it concentrates on the needs of women and is available to them throughout pregnancy and up to three months after the birth.

The work of the pals is supported by community midwives and midwifery managers; the midwives acknowledge the value of the support pals give to women. Regular meetings are held to keep community midwives up-to-date and the importance of partnership working is acknowledged. At the first point of contact with a pregnant woman, the community midwife completes a risk assessment form and the Pals in Pregnancy service has been included on this. It is planned to link pals into priority localities within the city, so they will work more closely with midwives, health visitors, Sure Start initiatives and other agencies in these areas.

Recommendations for practice

❖ That the Pals in Pregnancy service be offered to all women who fit the criteria outlined above.

❖ The service should support and continue to work in partnership with midwives and that strong links should be developed with health visitors, Sure Start and other voluntary agencies in the area.

❖ That Pals promote positive health messages in a sensitive manner.

❖ That Pals be linked to specific localities so that they can develop closer links with the midwives working in their area and keep up-to-date about the services available in the area.

❖ That the pals continue to receive in-service training to aid their personal development and enable them to offer a high quality service to their clients.

Conclusion

Evaluation has shown that the service has a positive effect and, contrary to expectations, the EPDS scores of service users improved postnatally. Despite its limitations, the EPDS is a useful tool for professionals to use.

The Pals in Pregnancy service works in partnership with midwifery, health visiting and local voluntary services to offer support to vulnerable pregnant women, living in disadvantaged circumstances. The aim is to improve the outcomes for mother and baby. The service is targeted at women who are most in need of support (DoH, 2003). Evaluation of the service has highlighted that it has increased access to primary care services, other agencies and improvements in mental health for some women. For the future it is planned to integrate Pals further into district localities and to continue to work closely with midwives and health visitors. The links with other groups such as Sure Start and voluntary groups will be strengthened to help ensure that all women who meet the criteria for referral are offered the service. The health promotion role of the Pals will be extended and the possibility of further training to enable them to act as peer breastfeeding supporters is being explored. As the service expands and develops, the confidence and skills of the pals grows; some of them have gone on to further education or employment and this is another sign of the success of the service.

Pals in Pregnancy is an exciting service that uses specially trained local mothers to provide peer support to disadvantaged pregnant women in Coventry. It employs women who know what it is like to face difficulties themselves when pregnant. Their role is to befriend and signpost women to services and empower them to take control of their lives. Pals do not tell women what to do, although they may advise women to contact their midwife if they have a problem. They promote positive health messages in a sensitive manner, for example, they will give women information on how to stop smoking or the benefits of breastfeeding. They will not deal with women's problems for them, although they will accompany them to appointments or help them to explain their problems. Pals support women to make their own decisions in a non-judgemental manner. At the end of the period of contact they aim to leave women in a position where they are more resilient and better able to care for their families. To do this they may help the woman to find other activities or groups, whether this is a mother and baby group, English classes or further education. Evaluation of the service has shown that the women who use it value the support they have received from their pal and state that it has made a real difference to them. They appreciate that their pal gives them a personal contact number and that the service is responsive and flexible.

References

Barrera M (1986) Distinctions between social support concepts, measures and models. *Am J of Community Psychol* **14**: 413–45

Bashiri N, Spielvogel A (1999) Postpartum depression: a cross-cultural perspective. *Primary Care Update for OB/Gyns* **6**(3): 82–7

Bewley C, Gibbs A (1998) 'It doesn't happen around here'. *New Generation Digest* **21**: 4–6

British Medical Association (1998) *Domestic Violence: a health care issue?* BMA, London

Bulmer M (1986) *Neighbours: the work of Philip Abrams.* Cambridge University Press, Cambridge

Cohen S, Wills T (1985) Stress, social support and the buffering hypothesis. *Psychological Bull* **98**: 310–57

Confidential Enquiry into Maternal Deaths (2001) *Why mothers die 1997–1999. The fifth report of the Confidential Enquiry into Maternal Deaths in the United Kingdom.* RCOG Press, London

Confidential Enquiry into Maternal and Child Health (2004) *Why mothers die – 2000–2002.* CEMACH, London

Cooper P, Murray L, Stein A (1991) Postnatal depression. In: Seva A, ed. *European Handbook of Psychiatry and Mental Health.* Anthropos, Zaragosa

Coventry Statistics (2004) Coventry Statistics. Available on line: http://www.coventrystatistics.org.uk (accessed 22 April 2004)

Cox J, Holden J, Sagovsky R (1987) Edinburgh Postnatal Depression Scale. *Br J Psychiatry* **150**: June

Coventry Statistics (2004) *Infant Mortality Rates 1995–2001*. Available online at: http://www.coventrystatistics.org.uk/content/themes/health/reports/Indicator_293/ visu (accessed 22 April 2004)

Department of Health (2000) *Infant Feeding Survey*. DoH, London

Department for Education and Skills (2001) *Making a Difference for Children and Families*. The Stationery Office, London

Department of Health (2003) *Every Child Matters*. The Stationery Office, London

Egeland B, Erickson M (1990) Rising above the past: Strategies for helping new mothers to break the cycle of abuse and neglect. *Zero to Three* **xi**: 29–35

Egeland B, Erickson M (1993) Implications of attachment theory for prevention and intervention. In: Parens H, Kramer S, eds. *Prevention in Mental Health*. Jason Aronson, New Jersey

Erickson M, Korfmacher J, Egeland B (1992) Attachment past and present: implications for therapeutic intervention with mother-infant dyads. *Development and Psychopathology* **4**: 495–507

Green J, Murray D (1994) The use of the Edinburgh Postnatal Depression Scale in research to explore the relationship between antenatal and postnatal dysphoria in perinatal psychology. In: Cox J, Holden J eds. *Use and Misuse of the Edinburgh Postnatal Depression Scale*. Gaskell, London

Hirsch B, Rapkin B (1986) Social networks and adult identities: profiles and correlates of support and rejection. *Am J Community Psychol* **14**: 395–412

Holden J (1994) Using the Edinburgh Postnatal Depression Scale in clinical practice in perinatal psychiatry. In: Cox J, Holden J, eds. *Use and Misuse of the Edinburgh Postnatal Depression Scale*. Gaskell, London

Mooney J (2001) The hidden figure: domestic violence in North London. Online at: www.womensaid.org.uk Domestic violence statistical fact sheet (accessed 23May 2004)

Murray D, Cox J (1990) Screening for depression during pregnancy with the Edinburgh Postnatal Depression Scale. *J Reprod Infant Psychol* **8**: 99–107

Murray L, Fiori-Cowley A, Hooper R, Cooper P (1996) The impact of postnatal depression and associated adversity on early mother-infant interactions and later infant outcome. *Child Dev* **67**: 2512–26

National Institute for Clinical Excellence (2003) *Antenatal Care: Routine Care for the Healthy Pregnant Woman*. NICE, London

Oakley A (1992) Social Support and Motherhood. The natural history of a research project. Blackwell, Oxford

Oakley A (1998) Experimentation in social science: the case of health promotion. *Soc Sci Health* **4**: 73–88

O'Donnell S, Fitzpatrick M, McKenna P (2000) Abuse in pregnancy — the experience of women. *Ir Med J* **93**: 229–31

O'Hara M (1994) Postpartum depression: identification and measurement in a cross-cultural context. In: Cox J, Holden J, eds. *Perinatal Psychiatry: Use and Misuse of the Edinburgh Postnatal Depression Scale*. American Psychiatric Press, London

O'Hara M, Swain A (1996) Rates and risk of postpartum depression: a meta-analysis. *Int Rev Psychiatry* **8**: 37–54

Onozawa K, Glover V, Adams D, Modi N, Kumar C (2001) Infant massage improves mother – infant interaction for mothers with postnatal depression. *J Affect Disord* **63**: 201–7

Price S (2003) Domestic violence. In: Squire C, ed. *The Social Context of Birth*. Radcliffe Medical Press, Abingdon

Schonveld A, Kingswell S (1996) *Improving Maternity Information — A Consultation Process*. Coventry Health Promotion Service, Coventry

Schumaker S, Brownell A (1984) Towards a theory of social support: closing conceptual gaps. *J Soc Issues* **40**: 11–36

Seeley S (2001) Strengths and limitations of the Edinburgh Scale. Online at: http://www.pndtraining.co.uk/articles/SRSB1.htm (accessed 19 September 2004)

Spencer N (2003) *Weighing the Evidence, how is birth weight determined?* Radcliffe Medical Press, Oxford

Yoshida K, Marks M, Kibe N, Kumar, Nakano H, Tashiro N (1997) Postnatal depression in Japanese women who have given birth in England. *J Affect Disord* **43**: 69–77

4

Inequalities in the outcome of pregnancy: understanding the role of access to care

Rachel Rowe

Introduction

Women from the most deprived backgrounds are up to twenty times more likely to die during or shortly after pregnancy than more well off women (Confidential Enquiry into Maternal and Child Health [CEMACH], 2004). Babies born to socially disadvantaged parents are more likely to be born small, premature and with health problems and are more likely to be ill or to die in infancy than babies born into more affluent families (Office for National Statitistics [ONS], 2004). As they grow up, poorer children are likely to be worse off in almost every aspect of physical health, compared to children from more well off families.

Families from ethnic minority backgrounds experience similar increased risks of ill health or death during and after pregnancy when compared with white families (CEMACH, 2004).

These inequalities in the outcome of pregnancy are striking and persistent and raise challenging questions for those working in maternity care. Are there ways in which maternity care itself contributes towards these inequalities? Do women from different social and ethnic backgrounds, for example, have equitable access to the best quality maternity care? Are there things that midwives and others working in maternity care can do to reduce inequalities in the outcome of pregnancy? To answer these questions it is important to understand the wider context of inequalities in health and the many factors that combine to produce social and ethnic inequalities in the health of pregnant women, mothers and babies. This chapter sets the scene for the rest of the book by exploring these issues and looking at the nature of social and ethnic inequalities in access to care. Finally, it explores what midwives can do to identify and tackle social inequalities as part of their work.

Understanding inequalities in health

Across the whole of society, people in lower socio-economic groups or living in areas of social deprivation experience poorer health outcomes and poorer ongoing health compared with people from more affluent backgrounds. There is increasing evidence that ethnic variations in health are also a consequence of socio-economic inequalities (Nazroo, 1999). Babies, children and mothers are no exception to this rule and are at particular risk because families with children are more likely to be poor than childless households (Department for Work and Pensions [DWP], 2004).

The main determinants of health, and of inequalities in health, can be grouped in a variety of ways, but it can be helpful to consider four main categories (*Figure 4.1*):

⌘ Material circumstances and associated health hazards in the physical and socio-economic environment.
⌘ Behavioural risk factors and barriers to changing personal lifestyle.
⌘ Psycho-social factors.
⌘ Access to and use of health care.

These influences on health cluster together, interact with each other and in many ways are difficult to separate. For instance, having a healthy diet is not simply a behavioural choice, but is also influenced by the availability of cheap, healthy food, within easy reach of where you live. Similarly, attending for antenatal care in good time is influenced by several factors: whether the woman knows when to attend; whether the hospital or clinic is easy to get to; whether the woman feels sufficiently 'in control' of her life to take up the services available, and so on. Despite this complexity, in order to appreciate the scale of these influences and to identify the part played by access to care, it is helpful to look at each of these categories separately, considering the experience of pregnant women and families in particular.

Physical and social environment

Families living on a low income are more likely to live in poor housing conditions (Revell and Leather, 2000). There is a wealth of evidence linking poor housing to ill health (see Best, 1999 for a good summary). For example, cold and damp homes contribute to a number of respiratory illnesses; accidents to children in the home are more common in disadvantaged households; poorly constructed and poorly repaired buildings are more prone to pest infestation, bringing with it an increased risk of transmission of infection, allergies, exposure to pesticides and stress. Individual deprivation is linked with environmental deprivation in other ways. Healthy food may be less available and may cost more in areas where poor people live (Macintyre, 1999). It can be particularly difficult to afford a recommended diet in pregnancy when living on benefits (Dallison and Lobstein, 1995). Poorer families are less likely to have access to a car and more likely to live in areas with poor public transport, yet live in areas with fewer or smaller gardens and fewer safe play areas, reducing children's access to safe play areas and exposing them to the potential dangers of playing in the street (Macintyre, 1999). Deprived areas are also more likely to have a higher volume of traffic than wealthier areas, exposing residents to a greater risk of injury and higher levels of pollution (Davis, 1999). The effects of poverty and social deprivation combine to reduce women's access to sources of advice and social support such as shops, health facilities, parks and friends and may contribute directly to fatigue — broken lifts, heavy shopping, more physically demanding jobs and so on (Graham, 1984).

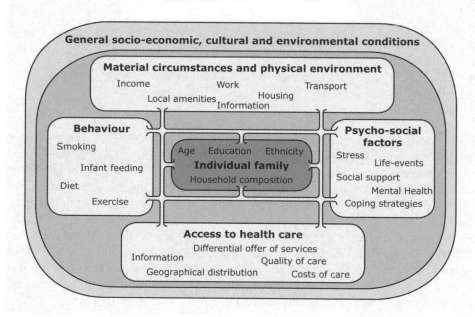

Figure 4.1: Main determinants of health

Behaviour

A range of health-related behaviours interact with these environmental factors to increase further the risk of ill-health in poorer families. In the UK, cigarette smoking is strongly linked to socio-economic status measured according to occupational social class (Rickards *et al*, 2004). Other indicators of disadvantage such as living in rented housing, lack of access to a car, unemployment and crowded living conditions are also associated with smoking (Wardle *et al*,

1999). In women with babies, smoking is also more common, both before and during pregnancy, in women from lower social classes, women who are unemployed or women who have never worked (Hamlyn *et al*, 2002). Hilary Graham has shown how smoking in women is inextricably linked with their caring responsibilities and their material and social circumstances (eg. Graham, 1987). The women who smoke the most are the poorer women, caring for more children, for children in poorer health and in an environment containing health hazards (Graham, 1994). The choices women make about feeding their babies are also associated with socio-economic status. Women from lower social classes or who have never worked are less likely to begin breastfeeding their baby and, if they do breastfeed, are likely to stop breastfeeding earlier than more well-off women (Hamlyn *et al*, 2002). Disadvantaged women may face greater barriers to choosing a healthier personal lifestyle because of a complex range of factors including lack of income, time or opportunity.

Psycho-social factors

Living in poverty is associated with increased exposure to severe life-events, such as serious illness or injury, job loss and marital breakdown. Studies of pregnant women and women caring for children at home show that working class women experience a higher frequency of life-events than more affluent women and that these life-events may be associated with increased risk of preterm birth and low birth weight (Brown and Harris, 1978; Newton *et al*, 1979; Newton and Hunt, 1984). Irrespective of severe life-events, women in lower social classes are more likely to suffer from anxiety, depression and phobias than higher social class women (Goldberg, 1999). Postnatal depression does not show a marked socio-economic gradient, but in disadvantaged households the effects of maternal depression on children's behaviour is more marked (Murray, 1997). Social support appears to have a protective effect in terms of mental health, acting as a buffer against stress and anxiety, but we have already seen that disadvantaged women may have reduced access to a range of potential sources of support.

Access to health care

Within health care, Julian Tudor Hart coined a phrase, 'the inverse care law' for the finding that medical care is least available where it is most needed (Hart, 1971). He was referring to the geographical distribution of health care and the phenomenon that healthcare resources are often found to be concentrated in prosperous areas, rather than in more deprived areas with the greatest concentrations of ill-health. However, even in the context of a healthcare system, where care is free to all at the point of delivery, other variations in access to care can still arise. Four reasons for variations in access to care are summarised in *Box 4.1*.

Box 4.1: Reasons why access to care may vary between population groups

Availability: Certain healthcare services may not be available to some population groups, or clinicians may tend to offer different treatment to patients with identical needs from different population groups.
Example: Women from some ethnic minority groups may not be offered antenatal screening because of an assumption by clinicians that they will not terminate a pregnancy so will not want screening.

Quality: The quality of certain services offered to identical patients may vary between population groups.
Example: Women who do not speak English are not likely to receive good quality maternity care if there are no interpreting and translating services.

Costs: The costs of care (financial or otherwise) may vary between population groups.
Example: The costs of attending antenatal appointments may be higher for poorer women who are more likely to be dependent on public transport. For women working in some low-paid jobs, the costs of taking time off work can be significant.

Information: The healthcare services may fail to ensure that the availability of certain services is known with equal clarity by all population groups.
Example: Clinicians may offer more information to articulate older middle-class women who appear interested in their care, compared to lower-class or young women who may be less confident about asking questions.

(Source: Goddard and Smith, 2001)

There are some aspects of health care in the UK where inequalities in access are apparent. Low utilisation of health promotion and preventive services, such as breast and cervical cancer screening and preventive health checks, is associated with deprivation at an area level and poor socio-economic circumstances at an individual level (Goddard and Smith, 2001). Dental health also shows wide class differences. Adults in non-manual occupations are more than twice as likely to report regular dental checks as those in manual occupations, and this may combine with different eating habits and care of the teeth to produce big differences in the proportion with no natural teeth (Drever and Whitehead, 1997).

Within maternity care there has been a general assumption that social class differences exist in the use of antenatal care and, at a local level, initiatives to promote access for particularly disadvantaged groups of women are widespread. Given the number and wide range of factors impacting on inequalities in health, it is apparent that access to care can only be part of the picture when thinking about inequalities in the outcome of pregnancy. It is, nevertheless, an area where there is potential for effective intervention. Given limited resources, it is vital that efforts to improve access to maternity care for disadvantaged women are appropriately targeted. It is important, for example, to establish whether there are particular groups of women who are more likely than others to book late for antenatal care or to miss antenatal appointments, and which groups these are, before setting up services aimed at improving antenatal care attendance. At a local level, requests for resources are more likely to be successful if they are backed up by convincing evidence of need. So, if we are concerned about social inequalities in maternity care, what kind of evidence should we look for?

The remainder of this chapter focuses on evidence of social inequalities in access to maternity care: what we know already and what midwives can do to find out about inequalities locally.

Access to maternity care

What does the research evidence say?

Evidence from other European countries and from the United States suggests that in those countries there are significant social inequalities in attendance for antenatal care. Being young, non-White, single or having a low income or low socio-economic status are all associated with starting antenatal care late or having a small number of antenatal visits (eg. Blondel and Marshall, 1998; Buekens, 1990; Delvaux *et al*, 2001; Essex *et al*, 1992; Roberts *et al*, 1998). A national survey in France also revealed substantial socio-economic differences in the likelihood of women being offered antenatal screening or women booking too late to be offered antenatal screening (Khoshnood *et al*, 2004). Given the potential impact of different healthcare systems it is not clear how generalisable these findings are to the UK so it is important to examine UK research evidence. Based on work carried out as part of a wider project looking at inequalities in maternity care for low-income and ethnic minority childbearing women, the research evidence on inequalities in access to maternity care in the UK is summarised in *Box 4.2.*

Box 4.2: Evidence on social inequalities in access to maternity care in the UK

Attendance for antenatal care

❖ *Evidence based on:* Systematic review of eight UK studies looking at the association between attendance for antenatal care and women's social class or ethnicity (Rowe and Garcia, 2003).

❖ *Quality of included studies:* Many studies were of poor quality or were poorly described and only one controlled for the effect of potential confounders such as age, parity or clinical risk factors. All but one were based on data collected between the late 1970s and the mid-1980s.

❖ *Findings:* Most studies found that women from manual classes were more likely to book late for antenatal care and/or have fewer antenatal visits than other women. Women of Asian origin were more likely to book late for antenatal care than White British women according to all four studies that looked at this issue.

❖ *Conclusions:* Although the available evidence suggests that there are social and ethnic inequalities in attendance for antenatal care, we cannot be certain because of the generally poor quality of the available UK research evidence in this area.

Offer and uptake of antenatal screening

❖ *Evidence based on:* Systematic review of nineteen UK studies looking at the offer and/or uptake of antenatal screening or diagnostic tests for pregnant women according to any measure of social class, educational status or ethnicity (Rowe *et al*, 2004).

❖ *Quality of included studies:* In most studies it was not possible to distinguish between the offer of testing and whether women took up the offer. Several of the studies were limited by small numbers of women overall or in some comparison groups. In many studies data, statistical analysis and classification of women's ethnicity were poorly reported.

❖ *Findings:* No studies found any significant inequalities in testing according to women's social class. Some studies suggested that women of South Asian origin might be up to 70% less likely to receive antenatal testing for haemoglobin disorders and Down's syndrome than White women. A small number of studies suggested that South Asian women might be less likely to be offered testing.

❖ *Conclusions:* Women from some ethnic groups, particularly South Asian women, may be less likely to receive antenatal testing for haemoglobin disorders and Down's syndrome. Significant

proportions of South Asian women will take up antenatal
testing if offered, but these women may be less likely to be offered
testing. The studies reviewed were not of sufficient
quality to rule out similar inequalities for lower social class women.

Dental care in pregnancy

❖ *Evidence based on:* One study of 500 mothers interviewed
within three days of the birth of their baby at Birmingham Maternity
Hospital in 1990 (Rogers, 1991). Women were asked about
their past dental attendance, attendance and treatment
during pregnancy, reasons for non-attendance. Socio-demographic
information was also obtained.

❖ *Findings:* Lower uptake of dental services in women in lower social
classes compared to more advantaged women. Muslim women
were also less likely to visit the dentist during pregnancy
than women with other religious beliefs. Non-attenders
during pregnancy were more likely to have been irregular
attenders previously.

Postnatal care

❖ *Evidence based on:* One study of 190 women in Oldham in the
early 1980s who were asked about their attendance for the
six-week postnatal check (Bowers, 1985).

❖ *Findings:* No significant difference in attendance rates between
social classes I, II and III (non-manual) and classes III (manual), IV
and V.

Attendance at child health clinics

❖ *Evidence based on:* Three papers on the subject of attendance
at child health clinics. These were all small-scale studies
carried out in London assessing attendance according to individual
measures of socio-economic status or area deprivation measures.

❖ *Findings:* In two studies using area based measures of deprivation,
mothers and babies from the poorest areas attended clinics more
frequently compared with families from more affluent areas
(Williams, 1981; Morgan, 1989). In one of these studies within an
inner city area individual social class was also associated with
attendance, with lower social class mothers attending more
frequently than mothers from higher social classes (Morgan, 1989)
In the third study, carried out in the late 1970s, visits to a child
health clinic were not related to individual measures of social class
(While, 1990).

Systematically searching for and summarising the research evidence in this way means that we can be confident about making evidence-based recommendations for policy and practice. The two systematic reviews and the summaries of other research evidence presented here are suggestive of social inequalities in access to key aspects of maternity care. In particular, they highlight the potential for social inequalities in attendance for antenatal care and access to antenatal screening, most notably perhaps with regard to women of South Asian origin. However, in many areas conclusions must be qualified because there are only a very small number of published papers or because the research that has been published is of poor quality. Furthermore, a number of key topics relevant to the issue of access to care are simply not covered by the research that has been carried out so far. These include, access for particular marginal groups such as very young women, women with disabilities, homeless women and substance-misusing women, and how language fluency and the availability of interpreting services affect access. So, given that the research evidence cannot answer all our questions about social inequalities in access to maternity care, what else needs to be done?

Tackling inequalities at a local level

Part of the process of doing a systematic review of research is to develop a clear question that you want answered by the review. You are then in a position to evaluate whether the papers included in the review enable you to answer that question and, if they don't, to make recommendations about what further research needs to be carried out to answer it. These recommendations can often be particularly useful for practitioners who want to answer similar questions about the services they provide. For example, in the case of the systematic review on access to antenatal screening, it was clear that to understand inequalities in access it was important to know whether inequalities arise because some groups of women are more likely to refuse screening, or because some women may be less likely to be offered screening in the first place. Because very few studies made this distinction, it was difficult to answer this question with any certainty. Findings such as these are summarised in *Box 4.3* and *Box 4.4* in the form of suggested approaches to finding out more about social inequalities in access to care at a local level.

In the first instance, these strategies focus on collecting evidence in a systematic way by carrying out an audit of routine data with regard to specific inequalities-related questions. As a preliminary step it is important to check sources of data to ensure that they are accurate and reliable. This process itself may be important in highlighting particular items of data that are not well-recorded or drawing attention to problems with the format of notes. Options for further work include carrying out more in-depth studies on particular groups of women, or on particular issues, such as staff training needs, changing services or setting up new services where necessary and evaluating any change.

Box 4.3: Tackling inequalities in attendance for antenatal care — suggested approaches

First steps: identify if there are inequalities in attendance for care

Carry out audit of maternity data system to find out whether women from some ethnic or socio-economic groups are more likely to book late, miss antenatal appointments or deliver without having antenatal care.

First, check your data sources — are the notes and records accurate? For example, did women recorded as delivering unbooked really have no antenatal care at all?

Suggested data items: maternal age; postcode (can be used to derive an 'area deprivation score'); marital status; ethnicity; primary spoken language; place of birth; occupation/partner's occupation (for individual measure of socio-economic status); gestational age at booking.

Could also compare perinatal health outcomes of women who book late/ deliver unbooked with women who book at recommended time.

Options for further work

1.   Find out more about reasons for late booking
Consider small scale qualitative research — focus groups or interviews – with late bookers or women who deliver without antenatal care to find out more about their reasons for booking late or having no antenatal care.

2.   Devise targeted intervention for groups of women more likely to book late
Consider community antenatal clinics, outreach services, etc guided by information from qualitative research.

3.   Evaluate
Use a simple before and after design, carrying out a repeat audit after your intervention has been running for a while.

> **Box 4.4: Tackling inequalities in access to antenatal screening — suggested approaches**
>
> **First steps — Identify whether there are inequalities in access to antenatal screening**
>
> Ensure that offer, uptake and refusal of screening are clearly recorded for each woman. Check your data sources — are records accurate? Carry out audit to find out whether women from some ethnic or socio-economic groups are less likely to be offered or to take up screening. Should also check whether some groups of women are more likely to book for antenatal care too late to take up screening.
>
> Suggested data items: maternal age; postcode (can be used to derive an 'area deprivation score'); marital status; ethnicity; primary spoken language; place of birth; occupation/partner's occupation (for individual measure of socio-economic status); gestational age at booking; screening offer; screening uptake.
>
> **Options for further work:**
>
> *1. Offer of screening*
> If some women are not being offered screening, consider why this may be. For example, is there evidence of ethnic stereotyping by midwives or other staff groups or language problems? Can you identify training needs for staff offering screening (see below)? Are there particular groups of women who are more likely to book too late for screening? Is there a need for specific antenatal outreach programmes for some groups of women?
>
> *2. Uptake of screening*
> Consider whether women have the opportunity to make an informed choice about screening.
>
> *3. Midwifery training needs*
> Consider whether there are professional barriers to women being offered screening. Are midwives sufficiently informed about screening policy? Are they confident in discussing screening tests with women from different social and ethnic backgrounds?
>
> *4. Consider appropriate intervention*
>
> *5. Repeat audit*

Conclusions

This chapter places the phenomenon of inequalities in the outcome of pregnancy in the context of the determinants of health more generally. This shows that the causes of social and ethnic inequalities in the outcome of pregnancy are many and complex. Access to maternity care is only one contributory factor, but it is important to identify where there are significant inequalities in access. Reviewing the research evidence in this area has helped to identify the questions to ask in order to identify inequalities at a local level, and has highlighted practical steps that midwives can take to tackle inequalities in their work.

Acknowledgements

With thanks to Jo Garcia, Maggie Redshaw and Andy Kirk for all their help.

References

Best R (1999) Health inequalities: the place of housing. In: Gordon D, Shaw M, Dorling D, Davey Smith G, eds. *Inequalities in health. The evidence presented to the Independent Inquiry into Inequalities in Health, chaired by Sir Donald Acheson*. The Policy Press, Bristol: 45–67

Blondel B, Marshall B (1998) Poor antenatal care in 20 French districts: risk factors and pregnancy outcome. *J Epidemiol Comm Health* **52**(8): 501–6

Bowers J (1985) Is the six-weeks postnatal examination necessary? *The Practitioner* **229**: 1113–15

Brown GW, Harris T (1978) *Social origins of depression: A study of psychiatric disorder in women*. Tavistock, London

Buekens P (1990) Variations in provision and uptake of antenatal care. *Baillieres Clin Obstet Gynaecol* **4**: 187–205

Confidential Enquiry into Maternal and Child Health (2004) *Why mothers die — 2000–2002*. CEMACH, London

Dallison J, Lobstein T (1995) *Poor expectations. Poverty and undernourishment in pregnancy*. NCH Action for Children, Maternity Alliance, London

Davis A (1999) Inequalities of health: road transport and pollution. In: Gordon D, Shaw M, Dorling D, Davey Smith G, eds. *Inequalities in health. The evidence presented to the Independent Inquiry into Inequalities in Health, chaired by Sir Donald Acheson*. The Policy Press, Bristol: 170–84

Delvaux T, Buekens P, Godin I, Boutsen M (2001) Barriers to prenatal care in Europe. *Am J Prev Med* **21**: 52–9

Drever K, Whitehead M, eds. (1997) *Health Inequalities. Series DS No.15*. The Stationery Office, London

Department for Work and Pensions (2004) *Households Below Average Income 1994/5 –2002/03*. Corporate Document Services, Leeds

Essex, Counsell AM, Geddis DC (1992) The demographic characteristics of early and late attenders for antenatal care. *Aust N Z J Obstet Gynaecol* **32**(4): 306–8

Goldberg D (1999) Mental health. In: Gordon D, Shaw M, Dorling D, Davey Smith G, eds. *Inequalities in Health. The evidence presented to the Independent inquiry into Inequalities in Health, chaired by Sir Donald Acheson*. The Policy Press, Bristol: 207–12

Goddard M, Smith P (2001) Equity of access to health care services: Theory and evidence from the UK. *Soc Sci Med* **53**: 1149–62

Graham H (1987) Women's smoking and family health. *Soc Sci Med* **25**: 47–56

Graham H (1984) *Women, Health and the Family*. Harvester, Brighton

Graham H (1994) Gender and class as dimensions of smoking behaviour in Britain: insights from a survey of mothers. *Soc Sci Med* **38**: 691–8

Hamlyn B, Brooker S, Oleinikova K, Wands S (2002) *Infant feeding 2000*. The Stationery Office, London

Hart JT (1971) The inverse care law. *Lancet* **1**: 405–12

Khoshnood B, Blondel B, De Vigan C, Breart G (2004) Socioeconomic barriers to informed decision making regarding maternal serum screening for Down's Syndrome: results of the French National Perinatal Survey of 1998. *Am J Pub Health* **94**(3): 484–91

Macintyre S (1999) Geographical inequalities in mortality, morbidity and health-related behaviour in England. In: Gordon D, Shaw M, Dorling D, Davey Smith G, eds. *Inequalities in health. The evidence presented to the Independent Inquiry into Inequalities in Health, chaired by Sir Donald Acheson*. The Policy Press, Bristol: 148–54

Morgan M, Reynolds A, Morris R, Allsop M, Rona R (1989) Who uses child health clinics and why: a study of a deprived inner city district. *Health Visit* **62**: 244–7

Murray L (1997) Postpartum depression and child development. *Psych Med* **67**: 900–4

Nazroo J (1999) Ethnic inequalities in health. In: Gordon D, Shaw M, Dorling D, Davey Smith G, eds. *Inequalities in health. The evidence presented to the Independent Inquiry into Inequalities in Health, chaired by Sir Donald Acheson*. The Policy Press, Bristol: 155–69

Newton RW, Hunt L P (1984) Psychosocial stress in pregnancy and its relation to low birthweight. *Br Med J* **288**: 1191–4

Newton RW, Webster PA, Binu PS, Maskrey N, Phillips AB (1979) Psychosocial stress in pregnancy and its relation to the onset of premature labour. *Br Med J* **2**: 411–13

Office for National Statistics (2004) *Mortality statistics. Childhood, infant and perinatal. Series DH3 no. 35*. Office for National Statistics, London

Revell K, Leather P (2000) *The State of UK Housing. 2nd edn: A factfile on housing conditions and housing renewal policies in the UK*. The Policy Press, Bristol

Rickards L, Fox K, Roberts C, Fletcher L, Goddard E (2004) *Living in Britain. No 31. Results from the 2002 General Household Survey.* TSO, London

Roberts RO, Yawn BP, Wickes SL, Field CS, Garretson M, Jacobsen SJ (1998) Barriers to prenatal care: factors associated with late initiation of care in a middle-class midwestern community. *J Fam Pract* **47**: 53–61

Rogers SN (1991) Dental attendance in a sample of pregnant women in Birmingham, UK. *Comm Dent Health* **8**: 361–8

Rowe RE, Garcia J (2003) Social class, ethnicity and attendance for antenatal care in the United Kingdom: a systematic review. *J Pub Health Med* **25**(2): 113–19

Rowe RE, Garcia J, Davidson LL (2004) Social and ethnic inequalities in the offer and uptake of prenatal screening and diagnosis in the UK: a systematic review. *Pub Health* **118**: 177–89

Wardle J *et al* (1999) Inequalities in health. In: Gordon D, Shaw M, Dorling D, Davey Smith G, eds. *Inequalities in health. The evidence presented to the Independent Inquiry into Inequalities in Health, chaired by Sir Donald Acheson.* The Policy Press, Bristol: 213–39

While A (1990) Child health clinic attendance during the first two years of life. *Pub Health* **104**: 141–6

Williams PR, Argent EH, Chalmers C (1981) A study of an urban health centre: factors influencing contact with mothers and their babies. *Child Care Health Dev* **7**: 255–66

5

Challenges midwives face when caring for asylum seekers

Jenny McLeish

Introduction

Being an asylum seeker in the UK is 'a situation, not an identity' (Burnett, 2002), and asylum seekers are an extremely heterogeneous group. Midwives encounter asylum seekers from many different countries speaking many different languages, with a wide variety of backgrounds, family circumstances and past experiences that create a range of challenges for midwives seeking to deliver optimum care. Some women arrive in the UK with their partner and other relatives; some reach the UK alone and may have left other children behind. Some are young teenagers. Some have personal experience of persecution, including torture and rape; some have fled following the abuse or murder of family members; some may have more generalised reasons for leaving their countries of origin, such as war, discrimination or poverty. What they have in common is the experience of the UK asylum system which, in itself, creates challenges for the midwives caring for them. This chapter will address two broad types of challenges: those posed by the physical, emotional and psychological impact of the refugee experience on women, and those related to women's status in the UK as an 'asylum seeker'.

What is an 'asylum seeker'?

The first challenge for midwives is to identify who among their service users is, or has been, an asylum seeker. The term 'asylum seeker' is sometimes used inaccurately to refer to any migrant to the UK, particular 'illegal' immigrants. It should be remembered that people from abroad may legally come to the UK for many different reasons, including work, study, tourism, visiting family members, marriage, or seeking asylum.

An asylum seeker is a person who has made an application to the Home

Office for refugee status, on the grounds that she is unwilling or unable to return to her own country because of a well founded fear of persecution, for reasons of race, religion, nationality, membership of a particular social group or political opinion. If her application is accepted she is described as a refugee, and she is entitled to live in the UK permanently. Sometimes an asylum application is refused but the applicant is granted the right to stay in the UK on a more limited basis known as humanitarian protection (formerly exceptional leave to remain).

The Home Office does not collect statistics on how many asylum seekers give birth in the UK, but an estimated 13% of asylum seeking women may be pregnant on arrival (Le Feuvre *et al*, 1999). It should be noted that a baby born in the UK to asylum-seeking parents does not have British citizenship.

The impact of the refugee experience on asylum seekers' health

Senior medical examiners from the Medical Foundation for the Care of Victims of Torture state that:

> *The health of asylum seekers is affected by many aspects of their experience, both past and present, including multiple loss and bereavement, loss of identity and status, experience of violence and torture, poverty and poor housing, and racism and discrimination... The asylum process is lengthy, complicated and intrinsically stressful, with the continual fear for the asylum seeker, until the process is complete, of being sent back to the original country.*
>
> (Burnett and Peel, 2001a)

They summarise some of the physical and mental consequences specifically for women as: vulnerability to sexual assault, sexual harassment, rape, poor health, depression, loneliness, and the stress of overwhelming domestic responsibilities (Burnett and Peel, 2001b).

Physical health

Two studies of refugee women and asylum seekers have shown that they have higher rates than the general population of miscarriages, some obstetric complications and perinatal mortality, but significantly lower epidural analgesia, oxytocin acceleration and episiotomy rates (Jones, 2001; Lalchandani *et al*, 2001).

Asylum seekers from some countries may have particular conditions that are less prevalent in the general UK population, such as HIV, and therefore need specific post-diagnosis support as well as specicalist care. The latest available figures (www.hpa.org.uk) show that 638 HIV positive women gave birth in England and Scotland in 2002, an overall prevalence of 0.14% of pregnant women, but rising to 0.53% in inner London. Although antenatal testing has greatly reduced mother-to-child transmission, a quarter of maternal HIV infections in London were undiagnosed before delivery. Three quarters of new infections contracted through heterosexual sex were believed to have been acquired in Africa, and 2.5% of women from sub-Saharan Africa giving birth in the UK were HIV positive. Although there is a higher concentration of people with HIV in London than elsewhere, the numbers of HIV infections being identified and treated outside London (the majority of which were Black Africans) rose nearly threefold during 1997–2002, coinciding with the policy of dispersing asylum seekers.

Asylum seekers from some African countries may have undergone female genital mutilation (FGM) and need tactful, gentle and respectful examination as well as accessible information about the implications for labour and birth. The organisation FORWARD (Foundation for Women's Health Research and Development), which campaigns on FGM, estimates that there are 86,000 first generation immigrant refugee or asylum seeking women and girls in the UK who have undergone FGM, and these numbers are increasing with the arrival of asylum seekers from Somalia, Sudan and Sierra Leone (Powell et al, 2002).

Many asylum seekers have been raped. (The Black Women's Rape Action Project [cited by Cowen, 2001] estimates that half of female asylum seekers are rape survivors.) Midwives should be aware that the pregnancy may be the result of rape. Even where it is not, pregnant survivors of rape and torture need very sensitive care, particularly around ensuring clear consent for any touching (for example, internal examinations may be distressing).

Real continuity of care, in particular one-to-one care throughout the pregnancy, is of enormous value to asylum seekers who are survivors of traumatic events, to avoid the distress of having to repeat an account of what has happened to a new person at each appointment. A further challenge to midwives is to keep on the right side of the line that divides necessary professional enquiry and human compassion from simple curiosity about a woman's past, particularly as some asylum seekers are unclear about the relationship between the health service and the Home Office and therefore what they 'have to' tell health professionals.

Finally, asylum seekers should be asked about domestic violence on the same basis as other service users. High levels of domestic violence were reported in a study of refugees in east London (East London and City Health Authority, 1997), but the common practice of relying on a partner to interpret at antenatal appointments may make disclosure very difficult, and the Confidential Enquiry into Maternal Deaths (CEMD) re-emphasises the importance of providing professional interpretation in this context (RCOG, 2001). Midwives need to be aware that asylum seekers may need considerable extra support if they do disclose domestic violence (Ditscheid). Many are frightened of contact with the police because of experiences in their countries of origin or fear of deportation. A woman may feel unable to leave an abusive partner if her asylum claim is dependent on him and will need independent legal advice about her immigration situation. Asylum seekers are also unable to make use of women's refuges because they are classed as having no recourse to public funds, and are therefore dependent on the National Asylum Support Service (NASS) to provide alternative housing.

Action points for midwives

❖   Prioritise asylum seekers for continuity of care, especially where they are survivors of serious trauma.

❖   Consider how to record sensitive information about past events or health conditions affecting the current pregnancy so that confidentiality is protected but other health professionals are readily aware of relevant facts without having to ask the woman to repeat her history.

❖   Make information on HIV, FGM and other conditions available in relevant languages and establish referral paths to specialist local or national support groups.

❖   Use professional interpreters and ensure that the woman's partner is not present for at least one antenatal appointment, to facilitate disclosure of domestic violence. Where domestic violence is disclosed, advise the woman to seek independent legal advice on her asylum claim and any NASS accommodation.

Mental health

Pregnant asylum seekers may come into the maternity services suffering:

> *An experience of profound loss… (which) creates special dimensions*
> *of need for pregnant women, with consequent impact on their*
> *physiological, psychological and social profile during pregnancy.*

(Kennedy and Murphy-Lawless, 2001)

Many asylum seekers describe feeling predominantly sad and anxious during pregnancy, overwhelmed by the practical problems of their situation and dwelling more on past events (which may include the violent loss of other children) than on anticipation of the future. Postnatally, many describe sitting alone crying endlessly, feeling extremely lonely and isolated and desperately missing the support of family members, especially their own mothers. Actual diagnosis of or treatment for postnatal depression appears, however, to be rare.

Most asylum seekers come to the UK having left behind all or most of their existing social networks. The task of forming new friendships is complicated by the transitory nature of asylum accommodation and by language differences both from the UK population and from other asylum seekers. Even women who are in the UK with their husbands can experience profound loneliness, because their cultural expectation is for female companionship and the husbands are out of the home with male friends. Refugee or asylum support groups can provide women with a safe place to relax and to meet both other asylum seekers and English people, but many asylum seekers are unaware that such groups exist. It is, however, important to remember that while some asylum seekers value the chance to talk to fellow asylum seekers who have experienced similar problems, others (especially those who have fled civil war or ethnic conflict) may actively avoid people from their country of origin, for fear of meeting someone from the opposing side, or may find it difficult to trust the strangers they have been thrown with by chance.

Some studies (Greater London Authority, 2001) have found that the incidence of mental disorders arising from insecurity, anxiety and depression increases after the asylum seeker has been in the UK for some time, so it is important to understand the impact of the asylum system on mental health. Asylum seekers are acutely aware of their own powerlessness within the asylum system and live in a state of chronic stress about the possibility of being refused asylum and being made to return to their country of origin; and for new mothers there is the added dimension of fear for their child's future. For some women, the constant humiliation of their treatment in the UK further undermines their self-esteem and pushes them towards a bleak despair. On the other hand, for some women, giving birth to a child brings comfort in their distress both because the practical needs of the baby distracts them from thinking too much about the past and because they no longer feel alone in the world: one woman whose relatives had been killed, including her three-year-old child, said of her newborn baby:

Before I was alone, but now we are a family. He is a whole family for me.

Some asylum seekers are detained in detention (removal centres) which are dedicated immigration prisons run on behalf of the Home Office. Asylum seekers who have been detained while pregnant or with a young baby describe very intense feelings of despair, profound loneliness, and a frightening powerlessness in their daily lives, even to the point of feeling unable to protect a baby from harm. Detention is indefinite and the reasons for being detained are often poorly understood by the detainee, creating a situation of chronic stress and uncertainty. One pregnant woman said:

Having a baby in here would be like asking a person to commit suicide.

Action points for midwives

❖ Be aware that asylum seekers are disproportionately likely to suffer from depression both antenatally and postnatally, and liaise with local mental health services and health visitors to ensure follow-up.

❖ Make contact with local refugee/asylum support groups, and local ethnic minority community groups, and signpost asylum seekers to them. Be aware of the cultural sensitivities of different groups so that the appropriate group is contacted.

❖ Encourage detained asylum seekers to make phone contact with the local visitors' group for social support.

Challenges related to the status of seeking asylum

The support system

Asylum seekers are not allowed to work and cannot claim state benefits. This means that unless an asylum seeker can stay with friends or relatives, once she has exhausted any money she has brought with her she has to turn to the National Asylum Support Service (NASS) for support and accommodation. If she is an unaccompanied minor (under eighteen) she will be supported by the local authority social services instead. A newly arrived asylum seeker is put into an emergency accommodation hotel/induction centre while her claim for support is accessed, and if she is entitled to NASS support she will then be 'dispersed' away from London and the south east (where most asylum seekers arrive) to long-term accommodation elsewhere. NASS financial support is approximately 70% of the adult rate of income support.

Since 2003, NASS support is only available to asylum seekers who make their asylum claim 'as soon as reasonably practicable' after arriving in the UK. In practice, this has meant large numbers of asylum seekers becoming destitute and is the subject of legal challenge under the Human Right Act. This restriction does not apply to asylum seekers with children, and although it applies in principle to pregnant women without other dependent children, in practice, a pregnant asylum seeker who is destitute can apply for support from the local authority instead.

An asylum claim can take many months or even years to be decided, and many initial refusals are reversed on appeal. When an asylum seeker's asylum claim is accepted, she is entitled to look for work and to apply for state benefits on the same basis as UK citizens. When an asylum seeker's claim has failed on appeal, it is expected that she will leave the UK and if she does not, she may be detained and then removed (deported). Women and babies can also be detained at other stages of their claim. Although families whose asylum claim has failed currently continue to receive NASS support up until they leave the UK, there are proposals before Parliament to remove this support from the parents and take the children into care if the family is destitute. Pregnant women without dependent children are not entitled to NASS support once their claim has failed, unless they are too advanced in pregnancy to travel safely, in which case they can receive 'hard cases' support from NASS.

The complexity of this system means that some asylum seekers who need maternity care will be living with friends and relations, some sleeping rough, some living in emergency accommodation hotels or induction centres, some in NASS-sourced long-term accommodation (hostels, bedsits and flats), some in local authority accommodation and some in detention/removal centres. In the future, some may be living in the proposed new accommodation centres.

Life in hotels/hostels

It is important for midwives to understand the circumstances in which asylum-seeking clients are living because this materially affects their ability to engage with the maternity services and to follow advice on self-care. For example, women living in full-board hotels are not given a food allowance if they have to miss a meal at the hotel in order to attend a maternity appointment. The food provided in the hotels and removal centres is described by women as unhealthy, poorly prepared, even disgusting, and many go hungry because they feel sick when they try to eat it and have no access to snacks. Women have blamed their very poor diet for small-for-dates babies and failure to produce enough milk to breastfeed. Some hotels fail to provide basic necessities: no cots, no clean bedding, no infant formula even for the babies of HIV positive mothers, nowhere clean to bathe the baby (most women have to share toilets and washing facilities with many strangers of both sexes, and the communal facilities are described as dangerously filthy, as well as unsafe due to sexual harassment). Single women usually have to share rooms which poses particular problems for HIV positive women trying to manage medication without disclosing their condition.

Financial support

Women who receive financial support from NASS (set at 70% of adult income support rates) live on an extremely tight budget which undermines their ability to follow standard advice on a 'healthy' diet for pregnancy, especially as familiar food from their own cultures may not be locally available and some do not have access to any cooking facilities. It is important that any advice given should be realistic; one asylum seeker who had raised three children in her country of origin lost confidence in a midwife who criticised her for boiling her fourth baby's bottles instead of buying a steam steriliser. Most asylum seekers greatly value practical help such as second-hand clothes and baby equipment.

Dispersal

The system of 'dispersing' asylum seekers away from London and the south east also creates challenges for health professionals, in particular, the difficulty of keeping in touch with women as they are moved on from place to place at short notice, which may cause screening test results to be lost (NASS will not disclose new addresses to health professionals whose clients have disappeared). A similar problem exists in the practice of detaining asylum seekers and subsequently releasing them without notice. There is considerable inconsistency in the dispersal of women in very late pregnancy: some are exempted from dispersal until after the birth of their baby, while others are dispersed very shortly before giving birth, but in neither case is the woman herself given the choice. Last minute dispersal sometimes means separating a pregnant woman from friends or relatives living near the emergency accommodation just before she gives birth, while in other cases the woman may be desperate to move on from the emergency accommodation to a settled address before having her baby.

Action points for midwives

❖ Check that the woman is receiving all the support to which she is entitled. If she is supported by NASS she should inform NASS of her pregnancy to receive an extra allowance of £3.00 a week. Four weeks before her expected date of delivery (or up to two weeks after birth) she can apply to NASS for a maternity grant of £300. If she is living in emergency accommodation she should receive £50 towards maternity necessities.

❖ Signpost asylum seekers to charities and support groups who can provide second-hand clothes and equipment; work with health visitors and local NCT or other mother-and-baby groups to encourage donations of second-hand goods.

❖ Be aware of the woman's accommodation situation and financial circumstances and tailor any advice accordingly; if she is in full-board accommodation try to schedule appointments to avoid conflict with meals or ensure that she is given some food.

❖ Be prepared to write a letter of support for women who need medical evidence to delay dispersal in late pregnancy or whose accommodation is unsuitable.

❖ Enable an asylum seeker's medical notes and test results to follow her when she is dispersed or otherwise moved, by supplementing hand-held notes with a pre-stamped change of address card for her to send to you when she finds out her new address.

Access to services and communication difficulties

All asylum seekers and refugees are entitled to free NHS health care, including community- and hospital-based maternity care. They have the right to be registered with a GP and pregnant asylum seekers are entitled to free prescriptions. Asylum seekers whose asylum claim has failed remain entitled to free community midwifery and health visiting services but not to non-urgent in-patient hospital care.

Entitlement to services is, of course, very different from having access to services. The challenges for midwives around access for asylum seekers can be grouped under three headings: physical access to services, communication, and overcoming negative attitudes.

Physical access to services

Although some asylum seekers become pregnant during their stay in the UK, others arrive in the UK with an advanced pregnancy and need to find out how to access the maternity services quickly. In particular, women who are unable to register with a GP need to be aware of the possibility of self-referral to the maternity services. In the past, women's information about maternity services has been primarily word-of-mouth from other asylum seekers, but there has been improvement in some areas with health screening at induction centres (Dover), or midwives holding clinics at emergency accommodation hotels (London). Pregnant asylum seekers also need information on how to reclaim fares to hospital using the HC1 form.

Pregnant women in detention centres should have access to normal maternity services, but they have to rely on the detention centre to take them to hospital appointments, which does not always happen.

Action points for midwives

❖ Work with the local providers of asylum accommodation and Home Office-funded One Stop asylum advice services to ensure that women at any stage of the asylum process have clear information on how to access the maternity services.

❖ Where there is a high concentration of asylum seekers using the maternity services, consider holding outreach clinics at their accommodation.

❖ Liaise with local detention centres to ensure adequate provision of maternity and child health services. Ensure the centres are aware of the importance of keeping hospital appointments.

Communication

Communication problems were identified as the key concern by providers of maternity services in a report on maternity care for newly arrived asylum seekers (Gaserud, 2001). In particular, community midwifery was felt to be compromised where there was no advocate or interpreter available, and midwives were dissatisfied with the language support available to women in labour, since advocates worked restricted hours and the language line interpreters working at night were usually male (Gaserud, 2001). That report described the situation in an area of inner London with a well developed advocacy service, but the Home Office policy of 'dispersing' asylum seekers around the UK means that the challenge of communicating with asylum seekers has been spread all over the country.

Changing Childbirth (DoH, 1993) recommends that:

> *Where (a woman's) first language is not English, interpretation*
> *facilities must be organised as early as possible and the woman*
> *given the name of a contact person who speaks her language... When*
> *a maternity unit is providing a service to significant numbers of*
> *women who are unable to communicate in English, it is essential that*
> *providers should develop linkworker and advocacy services.*

The CEMD (RCOG, 2001) reminds services of the importance of providing formal interpretation rather than relying on partners, children or friends. Women in detention centres may pose a particular challenge for arranging interpreters, as the centres often rely on fellow detainees for interpreting medical consultations or provide nothing at all.

There may be communication challenges at a deeper level than language. Midwives must remember that even experienced mothers are strangers to the UK maternity system and to the roles of different professionals within it, and many asylum seekers will not have access to antenatal classes to learn about what they can expect, due to arriving in the country too late or to language difficulties. For example, an area of frequent misunderstanding is the level of care available on the postnatal wards; many asylum seekers are shocked at the lack of practical help and support which would normally be provided postnatally by female friends and relatives in their countries of origin, and they benefit from thoughtful preparation on this point.

Asylum seekers' understanding of procedures and interventions may also be influenced by previous experiences of medical and maternity care in their countries of origin, and therefore extra care is needed to ensure accurate understanding of their options. For example, in the 'Mothers in Exile' study (McLeish, 2002) several women who developed high blood pressure described feeling very frightened about the prospect of induction or a caesarean, and experienced the decision-making process as one of coercion rather than informed consent. Many asylum seekers feel very vulnerable in their relationship with maternity professionals, especially if they have encountered negative attitudes; this may lead them to conceal concerns or questions and to attempt to be passively compliant in order to avoid attracting hostility. Asylum seekers, who often have complex information needs as well as feelings of powerlessness, may therefore particularly benefit from health advocacy.

Action points for midwives

❖ Identify a woman's language support needs at the first appointment, and arrange formal interpreting. Even where a woman prefers informal interpreting (eg by her partner), ensure at least one contact with her is without her partner.

❖ Consider provision of advocacy services. In any event, show genuine openness to questions and try to ensure that the woman feels able to express herself honestly.

❖ Liaise with the local One Stop service to identify any likely influx of particular language speakers to the local area, to facilitate planning of language support.

❖ Liaise with removal centres to ensure adequate interpreting support where needed.

❖ Give clear information about who the different professionals are and what they do, including what non-clinical support will be available (especially babycare support on the postnatal ward).

❖ Explain hospital procedures and potential interventions thoroughly, including the concept of informed consent. If possible allow interpreters to accompany women to antenatal classes.

It is impossible to overstate the importance to a woman living with the chronic insecurity inherent in the status of asylum seeker, of being treated decently by midwives. Warmth and kindness from midwives over the most apparently trivial matters can transform a vulnerable woman's experience of labour, and this is of enormous significance to asylum seekers who are disproportionately likely to give birth without a birth partner.

Unfortunately, many asylum seekers encounter hostility and racism from their maternity carers, including midwives, doctors, healthcare assistants and receptionists. This may take the form of explicit verbal abuse, or being made the butt of jokes by groups of midwives who are unaware that the woman can understand English. The challenge for all midwives is to create a climate of zero tolerance for racism within their service, to confront perpetrators, and to support women who are abused by colleagues in making a formal complaint. Forewarning an asylum seeker about negative attitudes she may encounter within the health service can also, to some extent, help her to cope with them.

> **Action point for midwives**
>
> ❖   Always challenge hostile or racist behaviour and comments by colleagues. Warn the woman about the possibility of meeting negative reactions and offer to support her in making a formal complaint if she does.

Support for fellow midwives

Providing care for a woman who has suffered extreme trauma, and who lives in very difficult circumstances can, in itself, be very stressful. A final and essential challenge for midwives caring for asylum seekers is to support each other, and to look after themselves as well.

References

Black Women's Rape Action Project (2001) Cited by: Cowen T *Unequal Treatment: Findings from a refugee health survey in Barnet*. Refugee Health Access Project, London

Burnett A, Peel M (2001a) What brings asylum seekers to the UK? *Br Med J* **322**: 485–8

Burnett A, Peel M (2001b) Health needs asylum seekers and refugees. *Br Med J* **322**: 522–47

Burnett A (2002) Speaking at the launch of the Department of Health's Information Resource Pack for Health Workers Caring for Asylum Seekers and Refugees

Confidential Enquiry into Maternal Deaths (2001) *Why Mothers Die 1997–1999. The fifth report of the Confidential Enquiry into Maternal Deaths in the United Kingdom*. RCOG, London

Cowen T (2001) The Black Women's Rape Action Project estimates half of female asylum seekers are rape survivors. Cited in: Cowen T, ed *Unequal Treatment: Findings from a Refugee Health Survey in Barnet*. Refugee Health Access Project, London

Department of Health (1993) *Changing Childbirth: Part 1. Report of the Expert Maternity Group*. HMSO, London

Ditscheid C *Refugee Women and Domestic Violence: The failures of state protection in the UK*. Available online at: http://www.refugeewomen.org

East London and City Health Authority (1997) *Refugees in Hackney: A study of health and welfare*. East London and City Health Authority, London

Gaserud A (2001) *Maternity Services for Newly-arrived Refugee and Asylum-seeking Women in the City and Hackney Boroughs of London.* City and Hackney PCT, London

Greater London Authority (2001) Cited in: *Refugees and asylum seekers in London: a GLA perspective, draft report for consultation.* Greater London Authority Policy Support Unit, London

Jones J (2001) *Refugees and Asylum Seekers in Enfield and Haringey: A health needs assessment/service provision review.* Enfield and Haringey Health Authority, 1999

Kennedy P, Murphy-Lawless J (2001) *The Maternity Care Needs of Refugees and Asylum-seeking Women: A research study conducted for the Women's Health Unit.* Eastern Regional Health Authority

Lalchandani S *et al* (2001) Obstetric profiles and pregnancy outcomes of pregnant women with refugee status. *Irish Med J* **94**(3): 79–80

Le Feuvre P *et al* (1999) *Asylum Seekers and General Practice: observational study of new arrivals in a Kent town.* East Kent Community Trust

McLeish J (2002) *Mothers in exile: Maternity experiences of asylum seekers in England.* Maternity Alliance, London

Powel R *et al* (2002) Female genital mutilation, asylum seekers and refugees: the need for an integrated UK policy agenda. *Forced Migration Review* **14.** Available online at: http://www.FMreview.org

Further reading

McLeish J (2002) *A Crying Shame: pregnant asylum seekers and their babies in detention.* Maternity Alliance, London

6

Female genital mutilation: consequences for midwifery

Anna Daley

There is little doubt that all women who undergo female genital mutilation (FGM) have a high risk of experiencing adverse outcomes. Midwives have a responsibility to be aware of the specific factors that will ensure that the care they give to women with altered genitalia is safe, informed and sensitive. It is, therefore, essential for midwives who have contact with this client group to have an understanding of the complex issues that surround FGM. The purpose of this chapter is to examine FGM and its consequences to women's health, particularly in relation to childbearing. The chapter gives midwives a fuller understanding of why it occurs, thus enhancing their practice and facilitating empathetic and appropriate care.

Female genital mutilation (FGM) refers to all procedures involving partial or total removal of the external genitalia or other injury to the female genital organs, whether for cultural or other non-therapeutic reasons. Its practice is known to persist across socioeconomic classes, and among different ethnic and cultural groups (Toubia, 1994; Momoh, 2000). FGM has no health benefits and can be fatal, complicating the already difficult task of childbirth and almost certainly causing some kind of physiological and psychological distress to every survivor (Graham, 1984).

Influential groups such as the United Nations (UN) and the World Health Organization (WHO) have condemned any form of female genital alteration and continue to work towards its eradication. WHO estimates that FGM is practised in approximately thirty African countries, the Middle East, parts of South East Asia and South America, and that two million young women are subjected to an act of FGM every year. This equates to approximately 6000 cases per day, or five girls every minute (WHO, 1993, 1995, 2000; Momoh, 2000).

The migration of people from cultures that practice FGM to Western societies has increased because of war, poverty and political unrest, creating a socially and economically marginalized refugee group. Healthcare professionals can be shocked, disgusted or even condemning when they learn their client has altered genitalia, a reaction that could be described as 'ethnocentric shock' (Stanton, 1995). This can lead to the further alienation of the client, as well as inappropriate care and intervention. These women can be fearful of healthcare professionals and have a poor uptake of healthcare services, and are often reluctant to disclose their condition to anyone outside their community (Momoh *et al*, 2001).

What is female genital mutilation?

Female circumcision and female genital mutilation are different terms used to describe the same thing, and both have become emotionally and politically charged (Royal College of Midwives [RCM], 1998). While mutilation is a strong term, it accurately reflects the harm inflicted and defines the act as a violation of human rights. The midwife, however, should be mindful of referring to mutilation in situations where it could cause offence.

FGM involves a variety of female genital operations that vary in severity depending on the amount of anatomic alteration that occurs (Shorten, 1995). FGM is most commonly performed on girls aged between four and ten years old, but can be carried out at any age, from a few days following birth, through childhood, adolescence and at times during marriage, pregnancy or childbirth, depending on the beliefs and traditions of the social group (RCM, 1998; Momoh *et al*, 2001).

FGM is usually performed by a female village elder or circumciser sometimes called a 'gedda', a traditional birth attendant who in some cultures is referred to as the 'daya', or a female family member such as an aunt, mother or grandmother (Mays and Stockley, 1983). FGM procedures are described in *Table 6.1*, are irreversible and have no known medical advantage (Dorkenoo and Elworthy, 1996).

Varieties of surgical implements used include razor blades, knives, pieces of glass and sharpened flints. Anaesthetic may not be used and the girl will need to be physically restrained. It is possible for her to lie with her legs bound together for many days following the circumcision and if the wound does not heal successfully she may be operated on again (Denholm, 1997). These factors, plus the skill of the operator, will affect the amount of scarring and damage caused to adjacent structures so, despite classifications, the type of mutilation may not be easily defined (Ahmed, 1996; Rushwan, 2000).

Table 6.1: Classification of female genital mutilation	
Type 1	Excision of the prepuce with or without excision of part or the entire clitoris (clitoridectomy). The removal of the prepuce is the only procedure which could be considered analogous to male circumcision
Type II	Excision of the prepuce and clitoris together with partial or total excision of the labia minora. The cut edges are then sutured together to leave a small opening
Type III	Excision of the external genitalia and stitching/narrowing of the vaginal opening (infibulation). During the operation a foreign body such as a slither of wood, is inserted to preserve patency for the passage of urine and menstrual blood once the wound is healed
Type IV	Unclassified. This includes pricking, piercing or incision of the clitoris and/or labia, stretching of the clitoris and/or labia, cauterization by burning of the clitoris and surrounding tissue, scraping of the vagina orifice or cutting of the vaginal wall and introduction of corrosive substances such as herbs into the vagina to cause bleeding

Why is it performed?

Humans tend to view the society in which they live as 'normal' and the unfamiliar beliefs and practices of other cultural groups as 'strange'. We use our society or culture as a measure to judge others. Sociologists call this 'ethnocentrism' (Stanton, 1995).

While people born and raised in a British culture will view FGM as incomprehensible and shocking, people who are brought up in a culture where FGM is an integral part of their society may view British culture as lacking morals and promiscuous. The Western culture's condemnation of FGM is often resented and seen as an unwelcome interference by practicing societies (Communicating for Change, 2002).

It has been suggested that the circumcision of women emerged from a patriarchal society with men needing to be assured that they were the father of their wife's children (El Saadawi, 1980). El Saadawi (1980) argues that the dominant classes and male-orientated social structure realized the power of female sexuality, which if unchecked could lead to confusion about the legitimacy of children and precipitate the collapse of the patriarchal family structure.

Other theories suggest that the most radical form of FGM, classified as Type III or infibulation, developed to protect the women of nomadic tribes against rape and to ensure their fidelity while the men were away from the group (Graham, 1984).

There are common characteristics shared by societies that infibulate girls. They tend to be patriarchal, with women in a low position with little political power, where men can demand a high dowry. Family identity and inheritance comes through the father's line and there is high male absenteeism as a result of polygamous marriages, war or men travelling away to find work. There tends to be the commonly-held belief that infibulation is a religious requirement and that non-excised women are religiously impure (El Saadawi, 1980).

Mothers see FGM as an important milestone in their daughter's lives, a marker of maturity (Booth, 1985).

Ahmed (1996) believes that infibulation is practised because it is a source of cultural identity that binds a community together.

Research among Somali women who had given birth in Canada identifies feelings of pride and purity about their circumcision, despite having suffered significant health complications and pain as a result of the infibulation (Chalmers and Omer-Hashi, 2000).

Within these cultures, there is a great deal of segregation between males and females. Sexual intercourse and genitalia are not discussed and women regard their genitals as belonging to their husbands and sexuality as a gift for reproduction, which is debased if discussed. They often do not expect to have any sexual fulfilment and have no concept of what normal female genitalia should look like (Mays and Stockley, 1983).

These circumstances do not encourage open debate. Even if the mother is strong enough to refuse FGM for her daughters, her children may still be at risk. There have been cases where small girls undergo FGM while in the care of their grandmothers, without parental consent (Mays and Stockley, 1983).

In 1998 the WHO estimated that as many as 50% of females in Nigeria have undergone some type of FGM (Momoh, 2000). Nigeria has the largest population of any African country, and the number of women who have undergone FGM equates to three quarters of the world's population of circumcized women (Hindley and Montagu, 1997). Many of the complex motives for performing FGM in Nigeria are shown in *Table 6.2*.

It is a common misconception that FGM is only performed by Muslim communities. The practice, in fact, predates Islam and is not mentioned in the Quran, although many practicing Muslims believe that there is a religious obligation to circumcise women (Schott and Henley, 2000). Uncircumcised women were considered 'dogs' by those who supported the practice in Nigeria (Communicating for Change, 2002). In Somalia, an uncircumcised woman is considered unclean and, therefore, unmarriageable. In these cultures, for many women marriage is the only option for them to lead fulfilling and significant lives. Being an outcast for these women is unthinkable.

Table 6.2: Motives for female circumcision in Nigeria	
Psychosexual	Reduction or elimination of the sensitive tissue of the outer genitalia, particularly the clitoris, so as to attenuate sexual desire in the female, maintain chastity and virginity before marriage and fidelity during marriage and to increase male sexual pleasure
Sociological	Identification with a cultural heritage, the initiation of girls into womanhood, social integration and the maintenance of social cohesion. There were also reasons associated with hygiene and aesthetic appearance, as some considered the external female genitalia to be dirty and unsightly and thought it should be removed to promote hygiene and provide aesthetic appeal
Mythical	Enhancement of fertility and promotion of child survival. It was found that some believed that if the baby touched the clitoris during child birth the child or mother would die, leading to clitoridectomy being performed during labour. There were those who considered the clitoris to be poisonous and a danger to the man if he came into contact with it. Another myth is that the clitoris would continue to grow if it is not removed
Religious	Female genital mutilation was found to be practised by people of various faiths (or no faith) in a range of communities. Most Nigerians that support the practice say it is because of tradition
Sources: Okonofua, 2000; Communicating Change, 2002	

Psychological considerations

The psychological needs and expectations of infibulated women are different and require specialized midwifery input to achieve a good outcome for mother and baby.

Although there has been little research into the psychological effects following FGM, the WHO regards psychological damage to women following this procedure as inevitable (Johnson and Rodgers, 1994; Momoh *et al*, 2001). Psychological trauma includes flashbacks, anxiety, depression, chronic irritability and reluctance to have sexual intercourse (WHO, 1996; Momoh, 2000). For these women the process of childbirth, with the need to expose their vulva and for that part of their body to be touched, can be deeply distressing and cause extreme psychological anguish (Schott and Henley, 2000).

Poor uptake of antenatal care by women with genital mutilation can mean their problems and concerns are not addressed during pregnancy (Chalmers and

Omer-Hashi, 2000). Cultural requirements, such as the woman being prohibited from bodily contact with a man other than her husband or the need to obtain permission from the husband or father before examinations can take place, will mean a woman is reluctant to be examined by a man, making routine antenatal care seem frightening and unacceptable. That fear is compounded when the woman does not speak English.

When living in a society that openly disapproves of FGM, it is common for women with genital mutilation to feel fearful of the reaction of healthcare professionals and be vulnerable to criticism. They may be embarrassed about exposing their genitals and may have heard stories about caesarean sections being imposed upon them or photographs being taken of their genitalia (Schott and Henley, 2000).

Midwifery care for women with FGM

The midwife must deploy specialist skills to ensure that sensitive and appropriate maternity care is provided to circumcised women. Implications for midwifery practice are summarised in *Table 6.3*. Any reaction of shock or disgust must be kept from the client and be dealt with separately by the midwife. She must reconcile her reaction with understanding so as to not blame the woman or her culture, and so that the woman's feelings and self-respect are 'considered at all times' (Schott and Henley, 2000). This reaction does not condone FGM but may foster a trusting relationship between midwife and client, which will improve health care, psychological status and outcomes for this group of childbearing women. These good relations could form the basis of education and support needed to eradicate FGM in the future (Graham, 1984).

The midwife should be aware of the ethnic groups who practise FGM, so that the subject can be approached at the first contact in pregnancy. For example, having established in the antenatal period that a woman has type III FGM, she should be advised that she will not be re-infibulated following a vaginal delivery. She may wish to be referred to a specialist clinic for further advice and counselling and will need to be informed as to what effect FGM will have on her pregnancy and delivery (Mwangi-Powell, 2001).

If a midwife is unsure of how to provide optimum care for a woman with FGM, she should refer her to a specialist clinic or, during labour, hand over her care to a colleague who is more experienced. The Foundation for Women's Research and Development (FORWARD) provides specialist study days to update practicing midwives.

Table 6.3: Midwifery care for women with female genital mutilation	
Consideration	**Implications for midwifery practice**
Terminology and phrasing	❖ Many women may not consider FGM an operation ❖ Reference to 'mutilation' may cause offence ❖ Discover how the woman refers to FGM herself ❖ Word question in an alternative way, eg. 'Have you been closed?' 'Do you have any problems passing urine?' A sensitive way of broaching the subject is suggested as: 'I know they practise female circumcision in your country, have you been cut or have you had circumcision performed?' (RCM, 1998)
English-speaking interpreters	❖ If the client cannot communicate effectively in English it is important an interpreter is provided ❖ The interpreter should be female, have good language skills with some knowledge of translation of medical terms and ensure the woman's confidentiality ❖ Make sure that the client, not the interpreter is in control and makes the decisions ❖ To ensure confidentiality, the woman and interpreter should not know each other socially ❖ The interpreter should not let her personal beliefs influence the way she translates ❖ It is not appropriate to use relatives or a child to interpret ❖ Visual aids and leaflets in the appropriate language will improve communication and mean the woman gains a clear understanding of the healthcare services and benefits that are available to her
Cultural sensitivity and privacy	❖ All healthcare professionals involved with the care of this client should ideally be female. Care by a male health professional can be seen as degrading or even sexually abusive and may be refused, even if the woman is dangerously ill. All men must be chaperoned ❖ Birth partners are likely to be female as traditionally men do not attend births ❖ It is usual for men to make all the decisions regarding their wife's care and must be included in this process ❖ Keep the number of people in the delivery room to a minimum ❖ Do not leave the woman exposed or uncovered for any longer than is necessary ❖ Informed consent should be obtained for those present and for any procedures performed
Pain relief	❖ The woman may not verbalise her pain and silence should not be taken as consent or a sign of tolerance for an examination ❖ Consider the use of a paediatric speculum or ultrasound imaging if a manual vaginal examination is not possible ❖ Epidural analgesia may prove the most effective form of pain relief during labour ❖ FGM can increase pain in the postnatal period and this requires appropriate management ❖ Perineal pain can have a significant effect on the success of breastfeeding

Physiology of FGM and its implications

There are adverse health outcomes and physiological complications with any type of FGM, but the most severe are associated with infibulation (Hindley and Montagu, 1997). The midwife should be aware that pregnancy and childbirth can exacerbate these problems, therefore appropriate labour management is essential to promote the physical wellbeing of the woman (Shorten, 1995). Complications can be grouped into three categories (*Table 6.4*):

* immediate
* intermediate
* long-term.

Table 6.4: Complications of female genital mutilation	
Immediate complications	❖ Extreme pain and shock ❖ Excessive haemorrhage and injury to adjacent tissues (urethra, rectum) ❖ Transmission of infection (HIV, hepatitis B, tetanus) ❖ Urine retention and subsequent urinary tract infections
Intermediate complications	❖ Delayed healing and scarring can lead to continued risk of infection ❖ Keloid scars (hard, prominent and irregular scar tissue) are inelastic and can obstruct the descent of the fetal head during childbirth, leading to prolonged labour and potential fetal hypoxia ❖ Development of recto-vaginal and/or vesico-vaginal fistula. Prolonged labour contributes to development of obstetric fistula when the fetal head applies constant pressure to the structures of the pelvis, causing necrosis of the vaginal wall ❖ Cystocele, or rectocele, cysts that develop in the urinary tract or digestive tract and predispose the woman to recurrent infection, pain and faecal and urinary retention ❖ Vulval ulcerations, abscess and neuromata
Long-term complications	❖ Dysmenorrhoea ❖ Endometriosis ❖ Recurring urinary tract infection ❖ Pelvic inflammatory disease ❖ Infertility ❖ Odour ❖ Painful coitus and impaired sexual response
Sources: Macpherson, 1992; Johnson and Rodgers, 1994; Shorten, 1995; Dorkenoo and Elworthy, 1996; WHO, 1996; Hindley and Montagu, 1997; Momoh, 2000; Rushwan, 2000; Mwangi-Powell, 2001; FORWARD, 2002	

Reversal of FGM, or de-infibulation

A reversal or de-infibulation can be offered to women with type III genital mutilation during pregnancy. Physiologically it is best performed at twenty weeks gestation, which allows time for the reversal to be completely healed before labour. The middle trimester may be considered a period of tranquillity for the pregnancy so a reversal is best performed during this time (Mwangi-Powell, 2001).

The advantage of de-infibulation before labour is that it allows access to the introitus and urethra during labour, which enables procedures to be carried out if that will ensure optimum care for the woman and her baby (Hindley and Montagu, 1997). Such procedures, if clinically indicated, include inserting prostaglandin gel, obtaining a high vaginal swab, artificial rupture of membranes, the application of a fetal scalp electrode or catheterization.

De-infibulation should be performed under adequate analgesia, including a general anaesthetic, and involves performing an anterior midline incision, usually along scar tissue, to expose the vaginal orifice and urethra. At times the clitoris is exposed when it has been buried under scar tissue (Momoh, 2000). The repair recreates a vulval opening by stitching over each of the raw sides so they do not appose. The suture material of choice is a fine polyglycolic acid suture such as Dexon or Vycril (Gordon, 1998). De-infibulation by laser vaporization is also an option and some research indicates that women prefer laser treatment as opposed to surgery despite the fact that it takes longer to heal (Omer-Hashi, 1994).

Episiotomy is likely for women with a significant amount of scar tissue so there is a risk that a woman who has already undergone de-infibulation would also need an episiotomy at delivery. Research suggests that some pregnant women who require de-infibulation prefer to have it done during the second stage of labour so that they only have to undergo one procedure (Momoh *et al*, 2001). There is some debate as to the optimum time for de-infibulation during labour. It can be performed during the first stage if requested or clinically indicated, although the favoured course of action seems to be making the incision as the head is crowning to keep the blood loss to a minimum and to reduce the chance of having both perineal damage and a wound from a caesarean section. With de-infibulation in the first stage of labour there is a risk that failure to progress, fetal distress, etc. could indicate a caesarean section. If it is carried out when the vertex is visible, there is a greater chance of achieving a vaginal delivery. Care must be taken not to damage the surrounding tissue or structures and adequate pain relief is essential (Hindley and Montagu, 1997).

De-infibulation at delivery should only be performed following appropriate and adequate counselling. Mwangi-Powell (2001) concludes that 'reversal in the second stage is unlikely to produce satisfactory results'. Gordon (1998) advises that if the woman presents in labour and is still infibulated, de-infibulation should take place in the first stage of labour and be performed by someone familiar with the procedure.

Micturition, menstruation and sexual intercourse will all be different after de-infibulation. For example, some women may think they have become incontinent following de-infibulation because of the significant increase in their flow of urine (Mwangi-Powell, 2001).

Physiological implications of FGM for childbirth

The anatomic alteration in a woman with genital mutilation leads to specific problems in childbearing. Antenatally, the structural change predisposes her to a higher chance of genitourinary infections and can also impede on diagnostic procedures such as collecting urine samples and obtaining vaginal swabs. Treatment with vaginal pessaries may not be appropriate (Hindley and Montagu, 1997).

In some cases, infibulation hinders internal examination so it is important for the midwife to build a calm, trusting relationship with the woman before any examination, and preferably before labour starts.

During labour, procedures (such as the artificial rupture of membranes, fetal blood sampling, the application of fetal scalp electrodes, catheterization or prostaglandin induction of labour) may be prohibited because of the severely reduced introital opening and the woman's deep anxiety and fear. Internal examinations should be kept to a minimum and midwives should be aware that, if permission is not granted by the appropriate male relative, an examination by a male healthcare professional may be interpreted as abuse by the woman or her family.

The woman should be encouraged to pass urine regularly during labour to avoid a full bladder (Hindley and Montagu, 1997).

The number of people in the labour room should be kept to a minimum and consent gained for those present. It is essential to have a professional interpreter if the woman is non-English speaking (Shorten, 1995; Schott and Henley, 2000).

Physiological difficulties relate to the scarring from the FGM procedure and the subsequent reduction in the introital size, and there is a risk of the rupture of scar tissue, extensive vaginal tears, rectal tears and haemorrhage (Johnson and Rodgers, 1994; Shorten, 1995).

Adequate pain relief throughout the labour is essential. As a result of the al   atomy, the pudendal nerve can be difficult to locate, making
)ck difficult to administer. During labour, the pain of the
             e re-stimulated, which may prove difficult to alleviate by any
             nalgesia. An epidural may prove the most effective form of
             1an, 1996). As with all labours, relaxation techniques, good
             d a trusting relationship with the midwife are important

contributory factors in pain management (Hindley and Montagu, 1997).

It is prohibited by law in the UK to re-suture the genitalia back to its previous state following delivery, as this is classed as re-infibulation, which even if requested by the woman or her partner, is illegal. Best practice is to sew over the raw edges as in the de-infibulation repair, but if consent is not given the edges should be left unsutured. As with all procedures, informed consent from the woman is essential (Momoh, 2000; Momoh et al, 2001).

The usual advice about hygiene, nutrition and pelvic floor exercises are applicable for women with altered genitalia during the postnatal period, but the main role for the midwife at this time is psychological support, with a focus on the altered anatomy and body image and referral to a specialist clinic if required.

Women with FGM have an increased risk of birth trauma such as bruising of the bladder and perineal injury, which will naturally slow the passing of urine in a woman who has impaired micturition. Adequate pain relief is important and will aid mobility, improve circulation and help to alleviate psychological distress.

The passing of lochia may be obstructed, making education about the symptoms of infection particularly important. Scar tissue can be slower to heal and postnatal care should include discussion with the couple about the resumption of sexual relations and family planning. The midwife should be aware that issues relating to sexual intercourse and female anatomy may cause embarrassment and should be dealt with sensitively, with the aid of a professional interpreter if necessary (Shorten, 1995; Hindley and Montagu, 1997).

Conclusion

FGM continues for a number of complex reasons involving issues of tradition, cultural identity, myth, moral codes and misconstrued information. It is not a requirement of any religion, although this is a common reason given for its practice.

A significant number of women who have undergone FGM now live and give birth in the UK, and these women have needs specific to the consequences of their altered genitalia. They require knowledgeable and sensitive midwifery care that is respectful not judgemental, understanding not intolerant, and enlightened not uninformed.

A number of groups and resources are available, which midwives can refer women to or can contact for professional support and advice. Improving communication and understanding will lead to improved outcomes for childbearing women and their babies. Midwives practising in an area where the number of circumcised women is high require specialist training to ensure that they uphold their duty of care.

The eventual complete elimination of FGM is the ideal, but in the shorter term the childbearing outcomes and experiences for women in the UK can be improved by healthcare professionals, providers and policy makers being aware and trained in the management of FGM and its complications.

Acknowledgement

This chapter is reproduced by kind permission of the *British Journal of Midwifery*.

References

Ahmed S (1996) Leaving the female body intact. *N Z Nurs J* **2**(4): 20–1

Booth E (1985) Building bridges across cultures. *Sister Links* **1**(2): 14–15

Chalmers B, Omer-Hashi K (2000) 432 Somali women's birth experiences in Canada after earlier female genital mutilation. *Birth* **27**(4): 227–34

Communicating for Change (2002) Uncut: playing with life. *CHANGES* **3**: 5–9

Denholm N (1997) Female genital mutilation. *N Z College of Midwives J* **17**: 5–16

Dorkenoo E, Elworthy S (1996) *Female Genital Mutilation: Proposals for Change.* Minority Rights Group, London

El Saadawi N (1980) Clitoridectomy: crime against women. *Spare Rib* **90**: 6–8

Foundation for Women's Health, Research and Development (2002) *Vesico-vaginal Fistulae (VVF). Facts about FGM.* Available online at: http://www.forward.dircon.co.uk/vesico.htm (accessed 20 August 2002)

Gordon H (1998) Female genital mutilation (female circumcision). *The Diplomat* **5**(2): 89

Graham S (1984) The unkindest cut. *Nurs Times* **80**(3): 8–10

Hindley J, Montagu S (1997) Midwifery care and female genital mutilation. In: Kargar I, Hunt SC, eds. *Challenges in Midwifery Care*. Macmillan, Basingstoke: 17

Johnson KE, Rodgers S (1994) When cultural practices are health risks: the dilemma of female circumcision. *Holist Nurs Pract* **8**(4): 70–8

Macpherson G, ed. (1992) *Black's Medical Dictionary*. A & C Black, London

Mays S, Stockley A (1983) Victims of tradition. *Nurs Mirror* **156**(21): 19–21

Momoh C (2000) *Female Genital Mutilation Also Known as Female Circumcision: Information for Health Care Professionals*. Guy's and St Thomas' Hospital Trust, London

Momoh C, Ladhani S, Lochire DP, Rymer J (2001) Female genital mutilation: analysis of the first twelve months of a southeast London specialist clinic. *Br J Obstet Gyaecol* **108**: 188–91

Mwangi-Powell F (2001) *Female Genital Mutilation. Holistic Care for Women. A Practical Guide for Midwives*. The Foundation for Women's Health, Research and Development (FORWARD), London

Newman M (1996) Midwifery care for genitally mutilated women. *Mod Midwife* **6**(6): 20–2

Okonofua FE (2000) *Female Genital Mutilation in Nigeria: dispelling the myths and building coalitions*. University of Benin, Nigeria

Omer-Hashi KH (1994) Female genital mutilation: perspectives from a Somali midwife. *Birth* **21**(4): 224–5

Royal College of Midwives (1998) *Female Genital Mutilation (Female Circumcision)*. Position Paper No. 21. RCM, London

Rushwan H (2000) Female genital mutilation (FGM) management during pregnancy, childbirth and the postpartum period. *Int J Gynaecol Obstet* **70**: 99–104

Schott A, Henley A (2000) *Culture, Religion and Childbearing in a Multiracial Society: A Handbook for Health Care Professionals*. Butterworth Heinemann, London

Shorten A (1995) Female circumcision: understanding special needs. *Holist Nurs Pract* **9**(2): 66–73

Stanton G (1995) *Introduction to Sociology*. Ashford Press, Southampton

Toubia N (1994) Female circumcision as a public health issue. *N Engl J Med* **331**: 712–15

WHO (1993) *World Health Assembly calls for termination of harmful traditional practice*. Press release of the 46th World Health Assembly. WHO, Geneva

WHO (1995) Λ Report of a Technical Working Group, Geneva, 17–19 July 1995. WHO, Geneva

WHO (1996) *Female Genital Mutilation: Report of a WHO Technical Working Group*. WHO, Geneva

WHO (2000) *Female Genital Mutilation*. WHO, Geneva

7

Challenges midwives face when caring for pregnant prisoners

Viv Gray

Introduction

Pregnant prisoners are a small, diverse and sometimes challenging group to care for. This chapter will look at the nature of the women's prison population, considering the special needs of women prisoners in general, and those of pregnant prisoners in particular. Health care, both by the prison service and the National Health Service (NHS), is discussed. Consideration is given to the needs of prisoners during pregnancy, birth and early parenthood. The special needs of foreign nationals, drug users and women who will not be allowed to retain custody of their infants will be discussed. A list of resources with contact details for statutory and voluntary organisations working with, or interested in, pregnant prisoners is included at the end of the chapter (*pp. 93–94*).

The population

Women prisoners comprise a small but increasing proportion of the prison population, climbing from 3.5% in 1993 to 5.2% in 2000 (Home Office, 2001), with an average population of 3,350 in 2000. Of these, approximately 22% are on remand, ie. either unconvicted, or convicted but awaiting sentencing. Only 31% of these women will receive a custodial sentence (Her Majesty's Prison Service [HMP], 1999). Most women (80%) receive sentences of less than a year (Home Office, 2001). The majority of female prisoners are held for drug offences (37%), theft and handling (20%) and violence against the person (16%) (Home Office, 2001). Greater proportions of women than men are given custodial sentences for theft and handling, drug and forgery offences, and pregnant women appear more likely than non-pregnant women to be given custodial sentences (Howard League, 1997).

Most women prisoners (66%) are mothers, an estimated 34% of whom are single parents. Fifty-five per cent have at least one child under sixteen; one third have a child under five. Whilst most are cared for by their father (25%), grandmothers (27%) or other family or friends (29%), 11% are in care, fostered or adopted. It has been suggested that these figures, which are reliant on self-reporting, may be underestimates due to the women not wanting their children taken away from them, and their lack of trust in prison medical authorities (Howard League, 1997). Women prisoners who are already mothers may find difficulty maintaining contact with their other children. This problem is particularly acute for Foreign Nationals, the majority of whom are held for trafficking, and whose children are likely to remain in their home country.

There is a broad consensus amongst prison, probation and social services, as well as campaigning organisations like the Howard League and the Maternity Alliance, that custodial sentences may not be appropriate for women who are not a threat to society (Maternity Alliance, 1997). This would seem especially relevant where they are the primary carers of a child or children. Unfortunately, magistrates continue to issue custodial sentences (HMP, 1999). This may be because alternatives to custodial sentencing, eg. cautions, tagging, or treatment programmes for drug users, while financially cheaper, are perceived as soft options, and not providing a sufficient deterrent.

Women prisoners may be held in women's prisons, women's wings of mixed prisons, or temporarily in any local police station. Some prisons, including Styal, Holloway, Askham Grange and New Hall, contain mother and baby units (MBUs), and women who expect to be prisoners at the time they give birth may be assigned to these units towards the end of their pregnancy. On average, women prisoners may expect to spend 26.3 hours each week engaged in 'purposeful activity' (work, education or exercise), and an average of 11.1 hours on weekdays and 10.8 hours at weekends out of their cells. The prison service aims to allow all women prisoners to have a bath or shower once a week (Prison Reform Trust, 1999).

Women prisoners may have a number of special needs in addition to their incarcerated state. They are ten times more likely than the general population to have spent time in the care of local authorities (20% and 2% respectively) (Home Office, 2001). This figure rises to 40–49% in young prisoners (Social Exclusion Unit Report, 2002). Half of women prisoners report having experienced abusive relationships, either physical (2/3) or both sexual and physical (1/3). Of those who report abuse, 40% were under eighteen at the time of the abuse, and an additional 22% report experiencing abuse both before and after their eighteenth birthdays (Home Office, 2001). Women prisoners have lower skills of reading, writing and numeracy than the general population (Home Office, 2001).

Prison may provide women with shelter from violent partners and intolerable living conditions. It can reduce her chances of contracting infection through prostitution and offers women the opportunity to receive regular health check ups, regular hours, meals and sleep (Wilson, 1993). The density of population and lack of privacy within prisons can mean that pregnant women receive a great deal of social support from the other prisoners. However, it may also provide a fertile setting for bullying and intimidation of vulnerable groups.

Within prisons, there are two distinct social worlds, prison officers and prisoners. Antagonistic stereotypes may develop between two groups because they do not and cannot interact as individuals (Jones and Fowles, 1984). Prisoners may extend this distrust to everyone who they perceive as having authority, and this can include midwives. This can lead to prisoners feeling unable to be open with their health carers about all aspects of their history. It would therefore seem prudent for healthcare providers to avoid becoming associated with the prison service, as this may prevent them from gaining the trust of the women in their care. However, some prisoners may develop a positive relationship with a prison service employee, for example, their personal officer. And a prison officer may have particular insights into a prisoner's needs or state of mind.

Healthcare needs of prisoners

Women prisoners are more likely than the general population to experience multiple health deficits, including asthma, epilepsy, high blood pressure, anxiety and depression, stomach complaints, period and menopausal problems, sight and hearing difficulties, kidney and bladder problems. The proportion of women prisoners who had received help or treatment for a mental or emotional problem in the twelve months before entering prison was 40%. They are particularly likely to have a personality disorder (50%), or a history of deliberate self-harm and/or suicide attempts (40%). Forty-one per cent reported some dependence on drugs in the year before prison (Home Office, 2001).

It is difficult to be sure exactly how many pregnant prisoners are held at any one time, as the prison service does not routinely collect this information. However, in their survey, the Howard League found 3–4% of women prisoners were pregnant (Howard League, 1997), whilst in their survey of young offenders, 10% were pregnant. It is estimated that 10–12% of pregnant prisoners give birth while they are in prison, and in 1998, the last year for which figures are available, seventy-eight prisoners gave birth (Howard League, 1999).

The prison service aims to keep pregnant women on 'normal location', *Table 7.1* (Howard League, 1997), unless they have other health problems, but may move those near the end of their pregnancy to one of the prisons with MBUs. They believe that pregnant women should not be alone at night but should share a room or sleep in a hospital ward so that there are people around to help if necessary. Pregnant prisoners should have a call bell in their cell (Prison Reform Trust, 1999).

In 1983, international guidelines on health care in prisons were agreed in Geneva (CIOMS, 1983), outlining the duty of health personnel to protect prisoners' physical and mental health and to treat disease to the same quality and standard given to people outside prison. In the UK, the High Court has confirmed that pregnant women in prison are entitled to expect the same careful standard of care as those at liberty, and this has been echoed by The European Convention of Human Rights. The Royal College of Midwives (RCM) has produced a position paper on caring for pregnant prisoners (RCM, 1996).

Healthcare for prisoners is provided by medical and nursing staff employed by the prison service. In 2004, the employer has changed to the NHS, following the model of maternity care for prisoners. Traditionally, care of pregnant prisoners has been very medically orientated, they receive very little in the way of social or

Table 7.1: Pregnant prisoners, 16 May 1997 (after Howard League, 1997)	
Prison	Number of pregnant women
Askham Grange	No information supplied
Brockhill	3
Bullwood Hall	1
Cookham Hall	0
Drake Hall	4
Durham	0
East Sutton Park	1
Eastwood Park	9
Highpoint	0
Holloway	(average number) 25
Low Newton	1
New Hall	4
Risely	4
Styal	8
Winchester	0
Total	60

nutritional privileges, and there is little conformity between prisons (Howard League, 1997). However, recently there has been a move towards partnership with the NHS for maternity care. This service was initially developed between midwives from Wythenshawe Hospital and Styal Prison (Scott and Blantern, 1998), and is now operational between many other prison-hospital partnerships.

Prisoners are unable to exercise choice about many aspects of their maternity care, including where to give birth. Many prisoners experience fear about receiving unequal treatment from midwives. It is still the case that a prisoner's access to midwifery care is mediated by the prison. In other words, a pregnant prisoner wishing to contact her midwife must first get the permission of an officer to use the phone.

Groups who traditionally do not access health and maternity services as effectively as the general population are over represented within the prison population. These groups are known to experience higher rates of complications in pregnancy, with statistically poorer maternal and neonatal outcomes (Confidential Enquiry into Maternal Deaths in the United Kingdom [CEMD], RCOG, 2001; Confidential Enquiry into Stillbirth and Deaths in Infancy [CESDI], 2001). Midwives may use their contact with women at this time not just to provide maternity care, but also to provide information about healthy lifestyles, health promotion advice, and referrals to other services as appropriate. Discussion of safe sex, contraceptive options and cervical screening programmes would seem to be particularly relevant. If services are sensitively provided, women may be encouraged to access other health services in the future. Care should be taken in the selection of written health promotion materials in view of the reduced literacy of many prisoners.

Good practice points

❖ Pregnant women are entitled to the same careful standard of care as other pregnant women.

❖ Pregnant prisoners are especially likely to have other unmet healthcare needs. As well as providing care for this pregnancy, midwives may be able to provide health promotion, information and support.

❖ Pregnant prisoners are likely to have reduced or absent literacy, so care should be taken in the selection of appropriate health promotion materials.

Antenatal care

The sort of accommodations which many women take for granted during their pregnancies, eg. small frequent meals, satisfaction of cravings, extra rest as and when required, may be difficult or impossible for pregnant prisoners to obtain. Midwives should be aware of these constraints, as well as of prisoners' general lack of access to fresh air and exercise; baths and showers; and privacy. Additionally, pregnant prisoners may lack access to written information either because it's not there, or because they can't read it.

Despite these constraints, women prisoners are more likely to experience a pregnancy which reaches term, and have heavier, healthier babies, than comparable groups of women who are not in prison (Wilson, 1993). It is suggested that this may be due to the regular, adequate diet provided in prison, as well as the prisoners' reduced access to legal and illegal drugs. Despite these findings, any conversation with a pregnant prisoner soon turns to their felt need for more and better food. It would be helpful for midwives to ascertain exactly what is available to pregnant prisoners in order to give appropriate dietary advice. Where there is a regular population of pregnant prisoners, it may be sensible to arrange for a review of their diet by a dietician. The midwife may also provide health education to the prison officers, as they may be unaware of the dietary needs of pregnant women.

Antentatal care may be carried out within the prison, or in clinics, either in the hospital or community. In order to meet her 'responsibility to ensure that the women she cares for have an appropriate standard of care at each stage of the pregnancy whatever the circumstances of their lives' (Dimond, 1999), it will be necessary for midwives working in hospitals near to women's prisons to make sure that their services for pregnant prisoners are as similar as those available to non-prisoners as possible. This may be achieved by developing links with the prison service (RCM, 1996), but the importance of consulting user groups should not be forgotten (Department of Health, 1993).

Where a regular pregnant population is experienced, standing arrangements will exist, or should be developed, between the providing NHS trust and the prison. A named midwife, or team of midwives, may be given security clearance, and may be able to negotiate access to keys in order to move easily through the prison. Where a prison with an MBU is located near a hospital, midwives will be visiting regularly to provide postnatal care. Where women are staying in cells within police stations, or in prisons where pregnant prisoners are only occasionally held, these arrangements may not be in place. In these situations, it may be more difficult to establish good links between local midwives and the prisons. However, as any maternity unit can expect to receive ad hoc prisoners from nearby police stations, they should have guidelines in place for the care of this vulnerable group. Prisoners who have already booked maternity care prior to imprisonment will have to transfer their care, and upon their release they will have to transfer again.

Although more antenatal care is now carried out within prisons, and restraints are removed during antenatal consultations in the community, they are worn from the time the prisoner leaves the prison until she is seated in the waiting area of the antenatal clinic. In addition, she will be accompanied by two uniformed prison officers at all times. The women may experience embarrassment about chains and officer escorts on antenatal visits, and feel judged by the women around them in the antenatal clinic.

Women prisoners may not know in advance about the dates of their antenatal appointments, in case they arrange for an escape party to meet them at the hospital. Prison officers should not be invited to attend medical or midwifery appointments unless the prisoner specifically requests this. Women prisoners are not allowed to have access to cash, so may be unable to make purchases of scan pictures. It would be kind, and not unduly expensive, for hospital trusts to donate the photographs to these women.

Prisoners who are thought at low risk of escape (usually those who have been convicted and received a short sentence, but not foreign nationals or those with a history of mental health problems or drug use) may apply for compassionate temporary release. If this is granted, they are released into the community for their antenatal appointments providing they return to the prison straight afterwards.

Where a regular population of pregnant prisoners is anticipated, antenatal groups may be held within the prison. These may be facilitated by midwives, or by childbirth educators funded by the education service. They can be an interesting contrast to community run antenatal groups, typically attended by women of varying gestation and parity, many of whom will smoke roll-ups throughout the sessions. Prisoners are entitled to payment for attending 'education' sessions, so midwives will enhance attendance at group sessions by ensuring that they are registered as educational sessions, and attendance recorded. Care should be taken with teaching materials to ensure that they are appropriate to the needs, skills and situation of pregnant prisoners. Where pregnant prisoners present intermittently, midwives may need to arrange one-to-one sessions to discuss preparation for birth and life with a new baby, as the presence of uniformed officers may be inhibiting to the group process within a community antenatal group.

It may be a particular challenge for prisoners, midwives, and prisons, where the prisoner has a pre-existing medical condition, eg. diabetes, which requires regular medication. The provision of medications in prison takes place in a highly supervised manner, and medications are taken in front of the person administering them. It can also be challenging when a prisoner develops pregnancy associated complications, eg. pre-eclampsia. Frequent hospital visits, or hospital inpatient stays place a great strain on the prison establishment. Where insufficient officers remain in the prison, prisoners are confined in their cells for longer periods of time. Despite this, if the woman's condition, whether pre-existing or pregnancy associated, cannot be managed effectively while in prison, the prisoner will need to be admitted to hospital.

Good practice points

* Pregnant prisoners experience lack of choice about diet, rest and exercise. Midwives should explore what is available to women locally and liaise with the prison if provision is inadequate.
* Establishing links with the prison can improve the services available to prisoners, however midwives should not forget to ask the women what their needs are.
* Maternity units should have guidelines in place for the care of pregnant prisoners.
* Officers should be requested to leave the room during antenatal consultations.
* Pregnant prisoners are not allowed to have access to cash. It would be kind to offer free access to services which pregnant women usually pay for, eg. a copy of scan photos.
* Attendance at community-based antenatal groups may be difficult. Institutions and individual midwives need to consider how best to ensure that prisoners can access the information and support usually provided by these groups.

Antenatal admissions

Women prisoners with health problems may need to be admitted to hospital earlier than women in the community because of the difficulty of managing their health needs within the prison system. Whilst an inpatient, the woman will be guarded by two uniformed officers at all times. However, unless a particular security threat is posed, she should not be chained at any time during her stay. Security risks should be discussed between the prison governors and hospital management.

Women prisoners may have strong preference about being held in hospital. In hospital they have access to privileges, eg. unlimited visitors and access to telephones, not available to them in prison. Conversely, they are under much closer observation in hospital, having two dedicated guards. They may also feel isolated, having little social interaction with other inpatients who are not prisoners. Their preference may not be related to the severity or otherwise of their medical condition, although prisoners, like other women, are generally very concerned for the wellbeing of their babies.

The Board

A woman prisoner who hopes to keep her baby with her after its birth must apply to the governor for a place on a mother and baby unit. Her case will be considered at a hearing, 'The Board', which the prisoner and her legal representative may attend. The Board is usually held in the last few weeks of a prisoner's pregnancy. Where she is received into custody late in her pregnancy, labour is premature, or the results of an appeal process are pending, the decision may not have been made by the time the woman presents in labour. Consideration is given to recommendations from a multidisciplinary team, which may include prison officer, probation officer, prison medical officer, liaison social worker, and other specialists previously involved in the woman's care. The decision is made by the governor of the unit. If she wishes, the woman may appeal against the decision to the Home Secretary.

The prison service has historically made decisions in relation to MBU places which do not comply with the Children's Act, but when Judicial Review has been requested of these decisions, the women have been given a place on a mother and baby unit prior to the judicial review. It has therefore not been clarified in law whether the prison service ought to be complying with this legislation in relation to unconvicted children. However, the Howard League in 2002 successfully challenged the prison service assumption that the Children's Act does not apply to convicted children (Howard League, 2004).

Because the prison cannot undertake to carry out an assessment of a mother-baby pair, wherever a woman's local social services department has any concerns about her ability to parent her child, the woman will not get a place on the mother and baby unit. Women who are currently drug users, and those who decline to have themselves and their babies randomly searched and drug tested, are also not able to take up a mother and baby unit place.

The possibility of a place on the mother and baby unit is an especially powerful inducement to conform, and pregnant prisoners may exist in a state of 'emotional limbo' (Kitzinger, 1999), waiting to find out whether they will be able to keep their baby with them after it is born. In order to take up her place on a mother and baby unit, the prisoner has to be willing to comply with the regulations of the unit. This includes agreeing to submit to searching of herself and her baby at any time, and undertaking to be drug free. She must also be willing to stay in her unlocked cell as requested.

If the woman is not offered a place on a mother and baby unit, she will be separated from her baby following its birth. Where no suitable person is known to the woman, or where it is thought that she will not be able to resume care for the baby upon her release, the baby may be fostered or adopted.

Intrapartum care

When a woman prisoner believes she is in labour, she informs the officers in prison, who control access to the telephone. The officers telephone the hospital for advice, or if birth appears imminent, call an ambulance immediately. Because the prison service is keen to avoid births in prison, women may arrive at hospital in early labour and wait on an antenatal ward for some time, accompanied, as always, by their two uniformed prison officers. Alternatively, prisoners may arrive in second stage. The prison service has a commitment to provide women officers where possible as escorts for labouring women. However, due to staffing shortages, this is often not possible. Where staffing problems are particularly acute, officers from private security firms, have been employed.

The Prison Service Regulations guidelines 37.141 to 37.144 discuss the security of labouring prisoners. These clearly discount chaining labouring women from the time they arrive at the hospital. If the woman is a category A prisoner (eg. terrorist), or at high risk of escape, alternative security measures should be taken (Birth Companions, 2002). However, it would be impossible for a prisoner to request this from an accompanying officer. Therefore, once the woman is in active labour, midwives should ask that prison officers wait outside the labour room. They should not be present at the birth unless the prisoner specifically requests their presence after they have left the room.

Women prisoners may not have access to their partner, or a friend or relative for a number of reasons. Partners and family may be estranged, in another prison, or live in another part of the country. Foreign nationals are especially likely to be unsupported in labour. Birth Companions was established in 1996 to provide support to women prisoners from Holloway Prison during the birth of their babies. They were established following the campaign to end the use of restraints for women prisoners in labour.

Whilst they continue to focus their service on Holloway Prison, they will endeavour to find a volunteer birth companion for any detained pregnant woman. They aim to meet with women antenatally to discuss her history, and her wishes for this birth. A birth plan is prepared and sent to the woman for approval. When the woman goes into labour, she calls the group, who endeavour to send a birth companion to meet her.

Simple comfort measures are provided throughout the birth, and afterwards the birth companion will take photographs of the woman and her new baby (prisoners are not allowed to have cameras or take photographs). They will also purchase a culturally appropriate meal for the woman following the birth, these can range from traditional Caribbean foods to Big Macs. The birth companions will continue to provide support to the woman throughout the early postnatal period.

Good practice points

❖ Labouring women should not be chained. Officers are obliged to remove chains from any prisoner if medical personnel request this.

❖ Prison officers should be asked to leave the room of a woman in labour. If the prisoner specifically requests their return, they should be allowed back in.

❖ Prisoners are not allowed to have cameras, and if they have no birth partner they may have no photos of their baby until their release from prison. If a camera is available it would be kind to offer to take some photos following the birth of their baby.

Postnatal care

Women prisoners who return to MBUs with their babies are likely to have a very different experience of early parenthood to women within the community. They are held in small cells, where the doors are never locked (because the babies are not convicted), but which they must not leave unless given permission. They continue to complain about their diet, which may not be adequate if they are fully breastfeeding. There are no published figures on breastfeeding rates within mother and baby units. The prison service appear aware of the importance of breastfeeding (HMP, 1999) but in practice exclusive breastfeeding seems difficult to achieve. The women feel under constant observation, having little privacy, and feeling enormous pressure to be perceived as good mothers. The close proximity of other mothers may be a very supportive part of the experience, and certainly it is difficult to imagine any new mother within prisons complaining of isolation. Because they are relatively pleasant areas of prisons, MBUs are always included in tours of prisons for visitors, and spending time there can feel a bit like being in a zoo.

Historically, women prisoners have been assumed to be 'bad mothers' and in 1960, courses were held in Birmingham prison for the 'training of neglectful mothers in child care and housecraft, instruction in planning menus, coping in the house and knitting' (HMP, 1999). Today, The Anna Freud Centre in London is running courses to help prisoners to understand and improve interactions with their baby. The course specifically explores issues around separation for women who will be handing their babies out to other carers when they reach the maximum age for the MBU.

Women prisoners are not entitled to maternity pay, and prisons appear to be exempt from the Factories Act, therefore prisoners return to work soon after their return to prison. The baby may accompany the mother to certain activities, or may be left in a nursery, staffed by trained nursery nurses. In addition to the financial pressures on the women, there is a feeling amongst officers that having women prisoners on the wing all day, rather than in work, education or treatment, can cause disruption, and that women are lazy if they do not return to work soon after their return. This is likely to have an effect on initiation and duration of breastfeeding. Women who have experienced a difficult birth may find it difficult to obtain enough rest.

Women prisoners' lack of confidence in their health carers can be particularly acute when they are concerned about their baby's health. Whilst their babies are registered with local GPs, they remain reliant on the prison staff, particularly medical and nursing staff, to gain access to their services. Where good relationships have been established between the women and her midwives, it may be helpful to continue postnatal visiting beyond the statutory minimum of ten days.

Mother and baby units may accept babies up to nine or eighteen months of age. However, sentence planning, which considers the best interests of the baby and mother, begins planning for their separation as soon as they are admitted to the unit. Women who expect to serve a sentence of less than eighteen months from their baby's birth — 80% if women prisoners receive sentences of less than one year (Home Office, 2001) — may be able to keep their baby with them for the remainder of their sentence. Where the sentence exceeds this, it may be felt that earlier separation will be more appropriate, especially as the mother and baby units for babies older than nine months are in open prisons, and women serving longer sentences may not be eligible for a place in an open prison. Prisoners may hand their babies out to family members or friends for visits for a few days, and short visits are often carried out in preparation for separation. Where no suitable family member or friend is available, the child will be placed in the care of the woman's own local authority.

Good practice points

❖ Midwives should ensure that the diet available to breastfeeding women is adequate for their needs.

❖ Midwives should be aware that women will be encouraged to return to normal activities within the prison as soon as possible, so women who have had a difficult birth experience should be given the opportunity to remain in hospital until they are ready for a return to full activity.

❖ Midwives should be aware that women with a remaining sentence of more than eighteen months will be facing the prospect of separation from their baby at some point in the future.

Special groups

Foreign nationals and asylum seekers

Prisoners in these groups are likely to be especially deprived. They are unlikely to have family or friends to provide them with cash, or maternity or baby clothes or equipment. Many may have been received into prison from airports without even a change of clothes. They do not have access to state funds, eg. child benefit, to help with the purchase of disposable items such as sanitary towels or disposable nappies, or 'luxury' items (like soap) from the prison shop. They are also likely to be experiencing the practical and cultural differences that exist between countries in their expectations of pregnancy and maternity care. If they are unsuccessful in their application for an MBU place, they may have no relatives or friends to take care of their baby.

Women who will retain custody of their children

A search in MIDIRS has not located any guidance for midwives when caring for women who will not retain custody of their children after they are born. It would seem reasonable to suggest that this will have an effect on a woman's needs during the end of her pregnancy, the birth and the postnatal period. It should be borne in mind that the prison service uses guidelines different to those used by social services in the community to determine the suitability of women to retain custody of their infants, and that most prisoners will not pose an immediate threat to their infants' safety. It is therefore likely to be appropriate for the mother-baby pair to remain together until the mother is ready to return to prison. The literature relating to bereavement around the time of birth may provide some guidance for midwives in the building of memories of their babies for these women (Stillbirth and Neonatal Death Society [SANDS], 1999). On their return to prison, women who have not been given an MBU place will return to the general prison population, however they are likely to have particular need for sensitive midwifery care in the postnatal period. Midwives may need to ensure that additional support is available, eg. from the community mental health teams, for this vulnerable group.

Good practice points

❖ Women who will not retain custody of their baby in prison are unlikely to pose an immediate threat to their baby. Each case should be considered individually to ensure that as many women and their babies as possible are kept together in hospital.

❖ Where a prisoner is to be separated from her baby, midwives should assist her in acquiring memories of her baby, in the same way as would occur following a bereavement.

❖ Midwives should ensure that women who are separated from their babies are carefully followed up in the postnatal period. Support from mental health specialists may be necessary for this group of women.

Drug users

A full discussion on the needs of pregnant drug users is beyond the scope of this chapter, and readers are referred to one of the specialist works on this topic (Siney, 1999). Midwives should be aware that pregnant prisoners are especially likely to be misusing legal or illegal drugs. However, imprisoned pregnant drug users are often very keen to discontinue their illegal drug use, as this will allow them to apply for a place on a MBU. Babies born to drug-using mothers may need admission to neonatal units to manage their symptoms of withdrawal. Where drug use is suspected, these mother and baby pairs should not be returned to the prison until it is clear that the baby has no symptoms of neonatal abstinence syndrome.

Conclusion

To provide culturally competent care to any group of women, it will help to have an awareness of important issues facing that group, and some of the factors which make pregnancy different for prisoners have been discussed in this chapter. Awareness of these factors must be balanced with the need to treat every woman as an individual and assess her own particular needs. Culturally competent care should not endeavour to provide the same services to all people, but should focus on meeting each individual or group's particular needs (Priest and Schott, 1996). Midwives may find that some or all of the issues raised in this chapter also apply to detained asylum seekers, and those detained in secure psychiatric units.

References

Birth Companions (2002) *Birth Companions Handbook*. Birth Companions, PO Box 33804, London N8 9GZ

Council for International Organisations of Medical Science (1983) *Principles of Medical Ethics Relevant to the Protection of Prisoners Against Torture*. CIOMS, Geneva, cited in Wilson, 1993

Confidential Enquiry into Maternal Deaths (2001) *Why mothers die 1997–1999. The fifth report of the Confidential Enquiry into Maternal Deaths in the United Kingdom*. RCOG Press, London

Confidential Enquiry into Stillbirths and Deaths in Infancy (2001) *Confidential Enquiry into Stillbirths and Deaths in Infancy*. 8th Annual Report. Maternal NS Child Health Consortium, London

Department of Health (1993) *Changing Childbirth: Report of the Expert Maternity Group* (Cumberledge Report). HMSO, London

Dimond B (1999) Pregnant women in prison and the law on human rights *Br J Midwifery* **7**: 5: 297–9

Goffman E (1961) *Asylums: essays on the social situation of mental patients and other inmates*. Anchor Books, Doubleday, New York

Her Majesty's Prison Service (1999) *Report of a Review of Principles, Policies and Procedures on Mothers and Babies/Children in Prison.*

Home Office (2001) *Statistics on Women in the Criminal Justice System*. Home Office RDS, 2001

Howard League (1997) *Pregnant and in Prison*. Howard League Information, London

Howard League (1999) *In the Best Interests of Babies? The Howard League submission to the Prison Service review of principles, policies and procedures for mother and babies/children in prison*. Howard League Information, London

Howard League (2004) *Advice, Understanding and Underwear; working with girls in prison.* The Howard League for Penal Reform, 2004

Jones K, Fowles AJ (1984) *Ideas on Institutions: analysing the literature on long-term care and custody.* Routledge and Kegan Paul, London

Kitzinger S (1999) Birth in prison: the rights of the baby. *Pract Midwife* **2**: 1: 6

Maternity Alliance (1997) *The Maternity Alliance Participtory Open Space Conference Report, 21 May 1997.* Maternity Alliance, London

Prison Reform Trust (1999) *Prisoners Information Book: Women Prisoners and Female Young Offenders.* HM Prison Service, London

Royal College of Midwives (1996) *Caring for Pregnant Prisoners.* RCM, London

Royal College of Obstetricians and Gynaecologists (2001) *Why Mothers Die. The United Kingdom Confidential Enquiries in to Maternal Deaths 1997–1999.* RCOG, London

Stillbirth and Neonatal Death Society (1999) *Saying Goodbye to your Baby.* SANDS, London

Schott J, Henley A (1996) *Culture, Religion and Childbearing in a Multiracial Society: A handbook for health professionals.* Butterworth Heinemann, Edinburgh

Scott L, Blantern S (1998) Mothers and Babies within the Prison System. *Br J Midwifery* **6**(8): 512–17

Siney C (1999) *Pregnancy and Drug Misuse.* Books for Midwives Press, Cheshire

Social Exclusion Unit (2002) Reducing re-offending by ex prisoners. Social Exclusion Unit Report, 2002

Wilson J (1993) Childbearing within the prison system *Nurs Standard.* **7**: 18 25–8

Worsley P (ed) (1987) *The New Introducing Sociology.* Penguin Books, London

List of useful addresses

Birth Companions
PO Box 33804
London N8 9GZ
www.birthcompanions.org.uk
Providing practical and emotional support to women who face giving birth whilst in prison.

Howard League for Penal Reform
1 Ardleigh Road
London N1 4HS
www.howardleague.org.uk
Working for humane and rational reform of the penal service.

Anna Freud Centre
21 Maresfield Gardens
London NW3 5SD
www.annafreudcentre.org.uk
Developing innovative psychotherapeutic treatments for children and adolescents with emotional and behavioural difficulties.

Women in Prison
3b Aberdeen Studios
22 Highbury Grove
London N5 2EA
www.womeninprison.org.uk
Concerned with the welfare and education of women in prison.

National Association for care and Resettlement of Offenders
169 Clapham Road
London SW9 PU
www.nacro.org.uk
Making society safer by finding practical solutions to reducing crime.

Her Majesty's Prison Service
HM Prison Service Headquarters
Cleland House
Page Street
London, SW19 4LN
www.hmprisonservice.gov.uk
Serving the public by keeping in custody those committed by the courts... looking after them with humanity and helping them lead law-abiding and useful lives in custody and after release.

The Home Office
Public Enquiry Team
7th Floor 50 Queen Anne's Gate
London W1H 9AT
www.homeoffice.gov.uk
Government department responsible for the prison service

The Prison Reform Trust
15 Northburgh Street
London
EC1V 0JR
www.prisonreformtrust.gov.uk
Aiming to create a just, humane and effective penal system.

Maternity Alliance
Third Floor West
2–6 Northburgh Street
London EC1V 0AY
www.maternityalliance.org.uk
Working to improve rights and services for pregnant women, new parents and
their families. Have a particular interest ion pregnant prisoners.

Association for Improvement in Maternity Services (AIMS)
Helpline 0870 765 1433
www.aims.org.uk
Campaigning and supporting organisation, particularly interested in pregnant
prisoners and mother and babies in prison.

8

Challenges midwives face when caring for women who experience domestic violence

Jane Morgan

Introduction

There is growing recognition nationally and internationally, that domestic violence and abuse is a phenomenon that impacts on the lives of women and their families. The reasons for this growing recognition are multi-factorial and, in contemporary Britain, have been shaped to a degree by empirical evidence obtained from crime reporting that has demonstrated prevalence of domestic abuse and the impact that this has on crime and community resources, which has forced it onto government agenda.

Domestic violence is a serious criminal, social and medical problem that has profound consequences, which can cause long-term damage to people's health, well-being and development. It is acknowledged that prevalence is often under reported, and whilst some epidemiological studies of domestic violence in Britain have found lifetime prevalence rates to be one in four women, the incidence of domestic violence in pregnancy is unclear, with reported rates varying from 0.9% (Sampselle *et al*, 1992) to 20.2% (O'Campo *et al*, 1994) depending on methodology employed.

Defining domestic violence

The fact that there is no universally accepted definition of violence against women may present difficulties for integrating this phenomenon into policy and practice in contemporary Britain, as evidence-based practice will be dependent on the quality of research within a defined concept. However, there are key definitions that have been used to inform policymaking and practice. The United Nations Declaration on the Elimination of Violence Against Women defines violence against women as:

> *Any act of gender-based violence that results in, or is likely to result in, physical, sexual or psychological harm or suffering to women, including threats of such acts, coercion or arbitrary deprivation of liberty, whether occurring in public or in private life.*

(General Assembly Resolution, 1993).

This definition acknowledges the gender-base roots of violence in society and how social mechanisms can force women into roles subordinate to men. The definition encompasses three main areas: violence in the family, violence in the community and violence perpetrated by society. United Nation's Children's Fund (UNICEF, 2000) in its report *Domestic Violence Against Women and Girls* defines domestic violence as violence that is perpetrated by intimate partners and other family members and is manifested through physical, sexual, psychological and/or economic abuse. It suggests that domestic violence is one of the most prevalent, yet relatively hidden and ignored forms of violence against women and girls globally.

In 1993 the Home Affairs Select Committee Report on Domestic Violence defined domestic violence as any form of physical, sexual or emotional abuse which takes place within the context of a close relationship which, in most cases, will be between partners who are married, cohabiting or ex-partners, with the violence from an adult perpetrator directed towards an adult victim. It highlighted the gender bias, the abuser being predominately male and the victim female. It acknowledged the long-term health effects and the other areas it impacted on, such as housing, education, and freedom to live without fear and that it was not limited to any particular social group or class, it occurred across the social spectrum. This definition has also been adopted by the World Medical Association (1996) and features in British government publications and health professionals' policies. Schornstein (1997: 1) further refines the definition to include, 'a systematic pattern of abusive behaviours, occurring over a period of time, that may become more frequent and severe, and are done for the purpose of control, domination and/or coercion'. Apart from acknowledging the physical, sexual and psychological abuse, she goes on to include the destruction of property and pets in the definition. This definition certainly gives a very clear picture of what domestic violence is and how it impacts on the entirety of women's lives.

Dobash and Dobash (1979) also highlight how domestic violence can vary in frequency and severity and the most commonly reported factor in motivating the perpetrator is to gain power and control over another individual by the use of abusive behaviour. The majority of such violence, and the most severe and chronic, is perpetrated by men against women and their children (Department of Health, 2000).

The Royal College of Midwives (1997), whilst agreeing on the nature of the abuse in its definition, further refines the definition of the relationship, as:

> *Perpetrated by a man against a woman whom he has, or has had a sexual relationship.*

The focus on the defined relationship which is, or has been a sexual relationship, demonstrates the controversy that exists when defining 'violence' against women and how participants in the debate use the same word for different phenomena. It may also have implications for how the RCM Position Paper on domestic violence (1997) is internalised by midwives and how they subsequently disseminate the principles of this paper into their clinical practice.

Prevalence

Apart from the difficulty of an agreed definition of domestic abuse there is also difficulty encountered when trying to obtain empirical evidence from those reporting domestic abuse. The Home Office acknowledges that statistics on domestic violence are understated as incidents are either not reported, or not disclosed in survey interviews. Although current notifiable offence categories are classified by type of offence, more detailed statistics are kept on homicide, and in 1997 the Criminal Statistics for England and Wales showed that of the 224 female homicide victims, 105 women (47%), were killed by partners or former partners, and of the 426 male homicide victims, 34 men (8%), were killed by partners (Crown Prosecution Services Inspectorate, 1998). Epidemiological studies of domestic violence in Britain have found lifetime prevalence rate to be one in four women (Lovenduski and Randall, 1993), and annual prevalence rates one in ten women (Mooney, 1993).

The biennial British Crime Survey (BCS) is a pivotal resource which informs Government policy as it provides data from residents in England and Wales about their experiences of crime, whether reported or not to the police. Its survey in 1996 of a nationally representative sample of 16,348 women found a lifetime prevalence rate of domestic violence to be one in four women aged sixteen to fifty-nine (Mayhew *et al*, 1996; Home Office, 1999). In 1996, the BCS included a computer-assisted self-interviewing (CASI) questionnaire designed to improve data collection and confidentiality and found that 4.2% of women said that they had been physically assaulted by a current or former partner in the last year, 5.9% of women had experienced physical assault and/or frightening threats and lifetime prevalence of domestic violence to be 26% for women (Mirrlees-Black and Byron, 1999). Recent BCS support the findings of the 1996 survey (Kershaw 2000). It is acknowledged that both men and women can be violent, however, the BCS has shown a clear gender pattern to crime. On the whole, women who experience violence, experience it from their partner or ex-partner in their own home, whilst men who experience violence are at most risk of violence from other men outside of their home. Men are motivated to use violence to gain control or power over another person whilst women are more likely to use violence as self-defence. Furthermore, women report continued or increased violence by the perpetrator following separation from their abusive partner, and also around times of contact with their children should this arrangement be in place following separation.

Domestic abuse and its process

Despite differences and difficulties in obtaining a universally accepted definition of domestic abuse, common features of all definitions include physical, sexual and emotional abuse from perpetrator to the other person in the relationship. Prevalence has demonstrated that men are predominantly the perpetrators and women and children the victims. However, we need to acknowledge that domestic abuse can occur in any intimate relationship, including female to male, and same sex relationships. How we talk about domestic abuse can influence people's perceptions, understandings and how they deal with it. The word 'victim' is a term used by the British legal system to describe a person who has experienced a criminal assault. In the context of domestic abuse, this term has been criticised as it implies passivity and doesn't portray the true image of having to deal with domestic abuse as part of daily life. The term 'survivor' has also been criticised, as this term infers that the woman has moved on from an abusive relationship, when in fact she may well still be in it. For midwives in the maternity services, where the focus of the care is the woman, it is important to avoid the use of words that describe and label women, which then go on to reinforce stereotypes, but to refer to women as 'women who are, or may have experienced domestic abuse'. The term abuse is a more accurate term than violence as abuse encompasses emotional, psychological, sexual, and even financial abuse, which is all part of an abusive relationship. The term violence conjures up an image of black eyes or a bloody nose and does not acknowledge that there are other forms of abuse a woman may be experiencing.

The British Medical Association (1998) summarises some of the characteristics of domestic abuse as physical violence such as punching, bruising, kicking, slapping, scalding, choking, hitting, knifing, murder. It can also be sexual, such as forced anal, vaginal or oral sex, sexual assault using implements, forced prostitution or taking part in pornography. Psychological abuse includes verbal abuse, humiliation and degradation, threatening behaviour, criticism, jealousy and possessiveness, destroying personal belongings, all of which can result in women losing their confidence, self-esteem, and generating thoughts that they are going mad. Financial abuse is another form of domestic abuse where finance is withheld from the woman, severely restricting her daily living and independence, with the additional stress of being financially dependant on the perpetrator and also having to suffer the consequences should she not budget or spend according to his dictate. It is important to appreciate that even though all acts of domestic abuse are not acts of violence, they still have a detrimental impact on women's lives and their health. Also, some of the acts of domestic abuse are criminal offences and this needs to be considered when working with women in abusive relationships.

The perpetrator

Abuse is not usually an isolated incident where a man loses his temper and lashes out, but it is systematic behaviour which follows a specific pattern designed to gain power and control over another person. Attempts have been made to describe the characteristics of the perpetrator (Walker, 1984; Dobash *et al*, 1996; Miller, 1995; Schornstein, 1997) and common features of the perpetrator cited in the literature include:

- traditional view of men's position in the family and society, ie. man is head of household
- exaggerated need to dominate
- violence may have been part of his own upbringing
- pathological jealousy
- hostility towards women yet emotionally dependant on women
- low self-esteem and feeling inadequate
- insatiable ego needs
- poor impulse control, including explosive and unpredictable temper
- need for instant gratification
- use of sex to punish or to enhance self-esteem
- guilt free — including belief that women provoke their behaviour so violence is justified
- objectifies women so it is acceptable to be violent
- closeness only to partner — poor relationship/social skills with others
- no awareness of intrusive behaviour
- escalating behaviour over time, especially if partner pregnant
- controlling through threats of murder or suicide if partner threatens to leave.

Gilchrist *et al* (2003) found in their study of domestic violence offenders on probation, several key characteristics emerged including personality psychopathology, negative early experiences, unemployment and alcohol dependence. Their research study identified two types of domestic violence

offender, the 'borderline/emotionally dependent' offender and the 'antisocial/
narcissistic' offender. The borderline/emotionally dependent offender maintained
stormy, intense relationships characterised by intense jealousy, high levels
of anger, high levels of interpersonal dependency and low self-esteem. The
antisocial/narcissistic offender was found to display hostile attitudes towards
women, low levels of empathy, and this group had the highest rate of alcohol
dependency and previous convictions.

A number of societal myths have developed over the years which only
serve to coerce with the perpetrator and keep domestic abuse hidden in society.
Myths such as 'she asked for it' or 'she drove him to it', are entirely unfounded,
it is the perpetrator who performs the violence, he is responsible for his own
actions. We would not condone violent behaviour in other relationships such as
manager and employee, doctor and midwife, lecturer and student, which would
be a criminal offence, so why would we sanction domestic abuse? Regardless
of where the abuse takes place, it is a crime against the individual. By gaining
insight into the process of a domestic abuse relationship, it helps us dispel the
common myths around domestic abuse and be better able to assist women
who find themselves in this type of relationship. Another misconception is that
women gravitate to this type of man, even after leaving a violent relationship.
There is no evidence to support this myth, women would not actively choose to
be in an abusive relationship. Entering into a relationship requires investment
of time and self and we often enter relationships filled with hope, aspirations
and dreams of what may be to come in the future. As the relationship develops,
apart from the emotional investment, there may well have been other domestic
and legal changes such as marriage, cohabiting, financial investment, children,
change in work circumstances, all of which impact on the boundaries and
commitment in the relationship. Coupled with an abusive relationship, where
the shift of power has meant that the man now has control and the woman has
experienced a loss of self-esteem and confidence, and may feel her life is in
danger, it is little wonder that she feels that she is not in a position emotionally,
financially, or physically to be able to terminate the relationship. She may also
feel partly responsible for what is occurring as the perpetrator may say it is her
behaviour that has evoked his abusive behaviour. Consideration also needs to
be given to the fact that for some women they may not want the relationship to
end, they genuinely care for this man and will say that they love the man but
not his behaviour. Ending a relationship, any relationship, requires insight, time
and energy and adopting a proactive stance to end the relationship and move
on. This may include practical considerations such as a house move, financial
upheaval, change in childcare arrangements. Practical considerations, along
with emotional trauma and societal influences, can place considerable strain on
an individual during this period. For those women in an abusive relationship
this is further compounded by her psychological state, domestic and financial
arrangements and, most importantly, her personal safety. On average, women
will experience physical violence thirty-five times before reporting to the
police (Mirrlees-Black and Byron, 1999). Often the police are the last resort

for women who will avoid police contact and may try other avenues of help first such as general practitioner, employer, community agencies. It is well documented in the literature that women are in greatest danger when they have just left the relationship so advising a woman to leave him, which is often a common response, would place her in greater danger. Leaving an abusive relationship requires specialist support and safety planning from the appropriate agencies in the community.

There is an assumption that domestic violence is more prevalent in the lower socio-economic classes, however, domestic abuse is prevalent in all social classes, ages, groups, and ethnic backgrounds. Evidence from the literature suggests that the highest reporting of domestic abuse is from women in the lower socio-economic groups, as these women with little or no income are more likely to use refuge facilities and public sector agencies for assistance and are therefore more likely to be 'counted' and included in research studies (Mooney, 1993). Therefore, there will be groups of women experiencing domestic abuse who are more visible to midwives in our community, but it is important to be aware that domestic abuse defies all boundaries and the only common risk factor is being female.

Domestic abuse and its impact on health

Domestic violence can impact on a woman's physical and psychological health and the awareness of such is becoming increasingly recognised as a public health issue. Women may experience physical injury, as a result of a violent attack or a sexual assault, which may be acute or have chronic consequences. Psychological injury can manifest in depression, anxiety, post-traumatic stress disorder and suicide (BMA, 1998). Whether the woman chooses to access the health services or not for treatment, it is well documented in the literature the nature and extent of the trauma domestic violence inflicts on the physical and psychological well-being of women (Bullock *et al*, 1989; Denham, 1995; Butler, 1995; BMA, 1998). Stark and Flitcraft (1996) found that women who had experienced domestic abuse were fifteen times more likely to abuse alcohol, nine times more likely to abuse drugs, five times more likely to attempt suicide and three times more likely to be diagnosed as depressed or psychotic compared with women who had not experienced domestic abuse. Attempts have been made to cost financially the impact of domestic violence to the health service, including employers' costs for days lost through employees' sick leave and absenteeism. Stanko *et al* (1997) in the London Borough of Hackney estimate the overall cost of domestic violence to the public agencies in the borough as being over £5 million in 1996.

Despite the government placing domestic abuse on its agenda and the formation of national, regional and local multi-agency initiatives since the early 1990s, health have initially been slow to respond and engage with domestic violence fora and other initiatives (BMA, 1998).

In 1997 the Government introduced, *The New NHS: modern, dependable* which declared a statutory responsibility for health authorities to improve the health of their populations (Secretary of State for Health, 1997). The Health Improvement Programme was the local strategy for improving health of which domestic violence, as a public health issue, was included. In 1998, eleven health action zones (HAZs) were established, and a further fifteen in 1999, in key geographical areas in order to provide a multi-agency approach to developing local strategies to improving health, with some focusing on domestic violence as a priority within their strategy.

In recognition of the impact domestic violence has on health, the Chief Medical Officer in his Annual Report (DoH, 1997) highlighted the implications of domestic violence for the National Health Service, which included accident and emergency services, maternity services, child and adolescent mental health services.

Alongside this government stance, some health professionals have attempted to address domestic abuse prevalence and its health consequences for women and their families, along with the cost burden for the National Health Service that this incurs, by formulating policy for each in their respective health professional groups.

The World Health Organization (2002) published the first comprehensive review of the global impact of violence which has been developed to raise awareness of the impact of violence on morbidity and mortality and to encourage a wider role for public health in response to violence. The report highlighted that domestic violence is a common problem worldwide, with results from forty-eight population-based surveys from around the world demonstrating that between 10% and 69% of women had experienced physical abuse by an intimate male partner at some point in their lives. The report acknowledges the difficulty in obtaining a clear definition of the problem, but argues that as violence is often predictable and preventable, there should be political commitment to work on the prevention of violence by creating and monitoring national strategies to work on violence prevention.

Domestic violence in pregnancy

The incidence of domestic violence in pregnancy is unknown, with reported rates varying from 0.9% (Sampselle, 1992) to 20.2% (O'Campo, 1994), depending on methodology employed in the research studies, which are predominantly American, Scandinavian and Canadian. There is very little published research in Britain as to prevalence and effects on pregnancy. Some studies suggest that pregnancy acts as a trigger to domestic violence to either begin, or exacerbate (Campbell *et al*, 1992; Stewart and Cecutti, 1993; Mezey, 1997). The nature of the violent attacks changes in pregnancy, with blows to the abdomen, breasts and genitalia more common (Hillard, 1985; Bohn, 1990). The incidence of domestic violence and serious sexual assault increases in the postpartum period, making both mother and infant more at risk (Hedin, 2000).

Hunt and Martin (2001) in their book, *Pregnant Women, Violent Men: What midwives need to know* report succinctly on the current research, with analysis of the literature, which highlights the impact domestic violence has on women in pregnancy and childbirth and why it occurs. Hunt (2001) draws on her own unpublished qualitative study which found that one in three women in her study had been subjected to domestic violence in pregnancy. They described the injuries they sustained during in-depth interviews with her. It was during the second or third in-depth interviews that the women chose to disclose, suggesting that there may need to be a trusting relationship for women to impart this information.

Violence during pregnancy has been associated with miscarriage, placental abruption, chorioamnionitis, stillbirth, premature labour, low birth weight (Shumway *et al*, 1999; Bacchus *et al*, 2001). Trauma to the abdomen in pregnancy can result in fetal fractures, rupture of the uterus, liver or spleen and can ultimately lead to fetal and or maternal death (NHS Executive, 1998). Further studies suggest that to cope with living in an abusive relationship, there is associated smoking, alcohol and substance misuse which have an impact on fetal and maternal health (McFarlane *et al*, 1996).

Although it is likely that domestic violence is severely under reported, it is thought to be more common than gestational diabetes and pregnancy induced hypertension, both conditions which are routinely screened for in pregnancy (Mezey and Bewley, 1997).

The report of the Confidential Enquiry into Maternal Deaths in the United Kingdom (CEMD, 2001) highlights the impact domestic violence has on women's health and states the responsibility health professionals have to care for and support these women and refer to the appropriate agencies in the community. Of the 378 women whose death was reported to the Enquiry, forty-five (12%) had voluntarily reported domestic violence to a health professional during their pregnancy. Eight of the women were murdered by their partners or close relatives, and of those, three of the murdered women were of either Indian or Pakistani ethnic origin. The report highlights the needs of women from ethnic communities and stresses the importance of not using family members as interpretators. It advocates the need for cultural awareness and sensitivity amongst midwives and obstetric staff. None of the 378 women in the report had been routinely asked about domestic violence. The report concludes from this that 12% is probably an underestimate. The report demonstrated that there was little or no help offered to the women concerning the violence that they reported. Whilst the occurrence of domestic violence is statistically high, and under-reported, Williamson (2000) highlights the fact that, at present, there are few needs assessment studies which identify domestic violence as a specific healthcare issue.

Health professionals' response to domestic violence

The Department of Health (2000) acknowledge that virtually every woman uses the healthcare system in Britain at some point in her life, and suggests that this offers an opportunity for a woman experiencing domestic violence to access help and support, especially if she does not wish to be involved with the police or criminal justice system. In its *Resource Manual for Health Care Professionals*, the Department of Health (DoH, 2000) state that for the NHS to respond effectively and appropriately the following must be addressed:

- raise staff awareness
- create an environment conducive to disclosure
- develop protocols for women and children who are experiencing/or have experienced domestic violence
- establish appropriate referral channels with multi-agency approach.

Prior to the publication of this document, the late 1990s witnessed responses to domestic violence and health from a number of the health professional bodies in the form of reports and policies. The British Medical Association, in their report, *Domestic Violence: a health care issue*, actively encourages the medical profession, 'to raise their awareness of the problem and develop strategies to identify and reduce health implications caused by this major public problem' (BMA, 1998: 3).

The Royal College of Midwives states that midwives are ideally placed to identify, enable and empower women who are or have been experiencing domestic violence, and state clearly in its Position Paper No19 (RCM, 1997) that every midwife has a responsibility to do so. However, there is currently no evidence available which supports this stance taken by the RCM: that midwives are ideally placed and that they understand their responsibility.

Scobie and McGuire (1999) demonstrate this in their quantitative study which utilises a survey strategy approach. They distributed a postal questionnaire to one hundred midwives across two maternity units and from the sixty-seven questionnaires (67%) returned, results showed that midwives knowledge of domestic violence during pregnancy was 'inadequate' (*sic*) and midwives do not feel adequately prepared to deal with women who have, or are experiencing domestic violence. Other groups of health professionals endorse this view. Davison (1997) highlights the evidence that domestic violence signifies a huge social and health problem, and yet it remains a low-key issue in nursing. Davison goes on to suggest that nurses should improve their awareness in this area by further training and support. Morgan (2003) conducted a quantitative study using a survey design from a sample population of nurses, midwives and doctors in an 'Obstetric and Gynaecology Directorate' in a NHS trust. Of the 147 questionnaires (56.54%) returned, 84 (57.14%) members of staff had never been taught about domestic violence and health consequences and fifty-four respondents (36.73%) had only received a minimal amount of teaching in this subject area. The results highlighted that, on the whole, staff receive minimal or no input on the subjects of domestic abuse and health during their original pre-registration education, nor in the future during post-registration training. Not surprisingly therefore, the majority of the respondents were unaware of the current statistics available taken from the British Crime Survey (Mirrlees-Black and Byron, 1999), and only seventeen respondents were aware that at some point in their lifetime, 26% of women, just over one in four, will experience domestic violence. Only five respondents correctly identified that a woman is assaulted, on average, thirty-five times before reporting to the police. Not only is domestic violence a process, but so too is disclosure and women will endure many episodes of domestic violence before disclosure. If staff beliefs and understanding are different to the women's lived experiences, this may have implications for the success of domestic violence policy in maternity settings. The study also highlighted staffs' own experience of domestic violence with lifetime prevalence rate to be 22%, similar to national statistic. Again, this can have implications for success of policy in practice as, currently, there is no policy of support for staff who may be experiencing domestic violence in NHS trusts.

Some health service trusts have attempted to respond to the national directives on domestic violence and health. A quantitative study by Marchant *et al* (2001) set out to explore current policies and practices in NHS trust maternity units in England and Wales using a postal survey strategy. All heads of midwifery or the midwife with expertise in domestic violence in that trust were sent the postal questionnaire. One hundred and eighty-three (87%) of the two hundred and eleven NHS trusts participated in the survey and results found that 12% had written policies for identifying women experiencing domestic violence, 30% had some form of agreed practice, less than half offered a woman an appointment on her own. There is considerable variation in England and Wales as to how the maternity services have addressed domestic violence and the implementation of policies and guidelines into practice. The authors concluded that there should be clear guidelines for identification and referral, training, audit and integration of domestic violence policies with child protection.

A common theme of the policies and guidelines formulated are recommendations to inform and promote what policy dictates as 'best practice'. However, currently there is no evidence to support that what is in the policy is in fact 'best practice', with further debate in the literature as to what constitutes 'best practice'.

Detecting domestic violence in the health service

Women's views on routine enquiry

Whilst there is an increasing awareness of domestic violence, the impact it can have on women's health and recommendations for health professional practice within the health service, there is an under reporting by women of their experiences. Various reasons for women not reporting domestic violence have been cited in the literature (BMA, 1998) and include:

- the emotional relationship
- fear of reprisals
- minimising experience and hiding it from family/friends
- pressure to remain in relationship (internal and external pressure)
- effect on children, staying or leaving
- financial dependence on partner
- nowhere safe to go
- unhelpful response from agencies
- lack of confidence making it difficult to make a clear decision.

Miller (1995) suggests that women do not disclose domestic abuse for fear of having their child removed from them and also the experience of 'dual trauma', whereby the woman is abused by the perpetrator then feels abused by the organisational system she has chosen to confide in because of the way she is subsequently treated following disclosure. In health professionals' policies this concept is never referred to as a legitimate concern for the women the very policies are seeking to help.

In a review of the literature published in 1996, Richardson and Feder concluded that from the literature, as the reasons for domestic violence going undetected in health practice were multi-factorial, doctors in general practice should routinely ask women if they are experiencing domestic violence. They further recommend that this practice be incorporated into national guidelines to improve women's care. However, a later study by the same authors, but part of a wider collaborative study, amongst 1207 women attending general practitioners in London found a similar prevalence rate amongst the women and, in addition, found that pregnancy in the past year was associated with an increased risk of violence. However, the authors in this study now conclude that although only one in five women objected to the idea of routine questioning about domestic abuse, at present there is an absence of evidence of benefit to women for routine screening for domestic violence in healthcare settings (Richardson *et al*, 2002).

In a study carried out in twenty-two general practices in Ireland, women who attended their general practitioner were asked to complete an anonymous questionnaire. Of the 1692 replies, almost two-fifths of the women had experienced domestic violence but very few reported being asked about it.

The authors concluded in their study that most of the women who had taken part favoured routine questioning by their practitioner and suggest that asking women about their fear of their partner and controlling behaviour may be one way of identifying those who are experiencing domestic violence (Bradley *et al*, 2002).

Bacchus *et al* (2002) conducted a qualitative study in order to examine women's perceptions and experiences of routine enquiry for domestic violence in a maternity service. A purposive sample of thirty-two women were selected from a much larger group of women who had taken part in a pregnancy screening study using the Abuse Assessment Screen (AAS) devised by McFarlane *et al* (1996). Of the thirty-two women in the sample, sixteen had experienced domestic violence in the previous twelve months, ten of those included pregnancy, six did not, and sixteen women with no history of domestic violence. Using semi-structured interviews as a method, the main outcome measures were women's views on the acceptability and relevance of routine enquiry of domestic violence. Although it is not possible to generalise findings from this type of study, Bacchus *et al* (2002) concluded that routine enquiry in the maternity settings is acceptable to women if conducted in a safe, confidential environment by a trained health professional who is non-judgemental and empathic, without time constraints and limited resources. The sixteen women who had experienced domestic violence all stated that they would not voluntarily disclose domestic violence in the absence of routine enquiry. The women in the study and the authors acknowledged that personal and professional qualities of the midwife will have an impact on the relationship formed which will impact on level, or any type of disclosure. It is important to remember that in this study the midwives involved had all been trained in how to administer the AAS, how to respond and how to refer to community services. They also had access to support and advice from the research team. This model of training and support is atypical of practice in the maternity services in Britain.

Findings from the same qualitative study reported that the women scored highly on the measures for postnatal depression and post-traumatic stress disorder (PTSD) (Bacchus *et al*, 2003). The study found that when seeking help from health professionals, the women found the general practitioner and staff in the accident and emergency department less helpful compared to the health visitors in responding to domestic violence. Emerging themes, such as lack of continuity of carer, lack of privacy and time constraints were a hindrance to disclosure by the women, which are consistent findings with other studies. The women reported that in the absence of direct enquiry regarding domestic violence, they were not inclined to initiate disclosure themselves. The authors conclude that although this is a small, descriptive study and not generisable, they suggest that health professionals should be prepared to initiate discussion about domestic violence and have sufficient understanding and knowledge about the subject to facilitate appropriate care for the woman.

A cross-sectional cohort study of 1500 women from five Queensland hospitals in Australia found that from the 1313 questionnaires (87.5%)

returned, 1286 (98%) believed it was a good idea to screen for domestic violence, although thirty women (2.4%) felt uncomfortable (Webster *et al*, 2001). However, there is no discussion in the paper as to whether the women who were recruited to the research had identified themselves in the antenatal clinic as having experienced domestic violence when asked by the midwife. Therefore, the prospective purposive sample of women may be biased to the non-abused group so they may not mind either way whether screening takes place. When asked which health professional should do the screening, multiple responses were possible, and 1068 women (64.9%) advocated midwives, 1055 women (64.1%) advocated general practitioners, 809 women (49.2%) selected social workers, and 771 women (46.9%) selected hospital doctors. Forty-two women (2%) said no one should ask. The authors acknowledge in their paper that the findings may be biased to those women from a lower socio-economic group, as the study only included women from the public hospital system and not the privately insured system. They suggest that their findings support other works that women do not mind being asked about domestic violence (Stenson *et al*, 2001; Caralis and Musialowski, 1997). They suggest that women believe the healthcare system to be a safe place to disclose domestic violence, yet their research questions did not address this concept, only who and when to ask the questions.

These studies widen the debate as to whether routine enquiry is acceptable in clinical practice. Women not included in the research study, ie. those who did not meet the inclusion criteria for the research sample, or those that did meet the inclusion criteria, but chose not to participate, may well be the very group of women whose voices need to be heard in order to inform policy and practice.

Health professionals and midwives

The Department of Health (2000) advocates that all health professionals need to be aware of the risks and impact of domestic violence on health, and be alert to the possible indicators that violence may be taking place, with appropriate support and referral protocols in place. The *Resource Manual for Health Care Professionals* suggests key questions that could be used for routine enquiry to take place in the maternity services (DoH, 2000: 25). The questions have been taken from a local multi-agency domestic violence forum, which has modified the abuse assessment screening tool developed and validated by McFarlane *et al* (1992).

'Good practice' guidelines have been developed by many of the health professional bodies, such as the Royal College of Obstetricians and Gynaecologists (Bewley *et al*, 1997), community practitioners (Peckover, 2001), Royal College of Midwives (1997), Royal College of Nursing (2000) and the Department of Health (2000). All advocate training and education for healthcare professionals and all are of the unanimous opinion that each healthcare worker, as an individual and collectively as a profession, has a responsibility to incorporate routine questioning about domestic violence into their practice. This is reflected in all the guidelines which advocate the use of routine screening to identify cases of domestic violence and the development of policy to deal with screening and disclosure. However, whilst all the guidelines appear to be evidence-based, drawing on evidence which demonstrates prevalence and health impact, there appears to be a paucity of research which reflects the voices of the women who have experienced abuse informing the policy and practice guidelines. The National Institute for Clinical Excellence (NICE) published 'Antenatal Care. Routine care for the healthy pregnant woman. Clinical guideline 6', in 2003 and states that healthcare professionals need to be alert to the signs and symptoms of domestic violence; offering women the opportunity to disclose in an environment in which they feel secure. This recommendation has been informed by only grade D evidence, and suggests that staff refer to the Department of Health publication, *Domestic Violence: A Resource Manual for Health Care Professionals* (2000).

A tension now exists in clinical practice whereby policy is advocating that healthcare professionals should incorporate routine enquiry into their clinical practice, yet training and support for staff is dependent on a trust's or primary care trust commitment to this issue.

Failure of health professionals to identify domestic violence and offer appropriate intervention has been documented in a number of studies (Brown, Lent and Sas 1993; Sugg and Inui, 1992) and includes reasons such as:

- inadequate knowledge and lack of training
- lack of time
- fear of offending the woman
- fear of opening a 'Pandora's Box'
- feeling powerless to 'fix' it for the woman
- belief that it is not their remit.

Morgan (2003) found that the trust where she undertook her research study did have a domestic violence strategy in place for the women accessing the maternity and gynaecology services to disclose domestic violence, but from the staff response, the women had never used this strategy. This is a clear example of policy formulation being developed without consulting the staff who would be responsible for implementing it, or the women for whom it is in place.

Ramsay *et al* (2002) conducted a systematic review of published quantitative studies in order to assess the evidence for the acceptability and effectiveness of screening women for domestic violence in healthcare settings. Twenty papers met the inclusion criteria. The authors concluded that screening by health professionals' increases the identification of domestic violence and most women do not object to being asked. However, most health professionals do not agree with routine screening in health. The authors acknowledged that although domestic violence is a common problem with health consequences, there is currently insufficient evidence to show whether screening and intervention can lead to improved outcomes for women identified as abused. This paper, published in a reputable medical journal, with a wide medical target audience, generated considerable dialogue among those in health and those with an interest or commitment to working in this field. Criticism of the paper included the nature of the studies included, ie. only scientific quantitative papers, the lack of grey literature, the fact that research studies are only beginning to emerge, the lack of acknowledgment of the complexity of work with domestic violence. Ramsay *et al* (2002) responded to some of this dialogue and suggested that as it is currently not known if screening does have adverse consequences for abused women, ie. inappropriate pressure to leave an abused relationship, then training is needed for staff on how to respond to women, including referrals to other agencies.

In the same journal, Taket *et al* (2003) published a response to Ramsay *et al* and firstly debated the feasibility of 'screening' for domestic violence in health: screening being the application of a standardised test or question according to a procedure that does not vary from place to place, with a standardised response. Asking about domestic violence does not fit this approach and Taket *et al* (2003) suggest that routine enquiry is a more appropriate approach. They go on to defend routine enquiry, despite the paucity of research which measures women-centred outcomes of health-based interventions and the fact that routine enquiry is not a proven intervention for women's health. They suggest that it should be part of healthcare practice as it enables health professionals to help women access further support, even though some staff do not wish to undertake this as part of their role.

As well as policy development at a national level for midwives (RCM, 1997), maternity units have forged ahead and developed local policy and strategies in an attempt to incorporate routine enquiry for domestic violence in maternity settings. Those initiatives published demonstrate similarities to the RCM Position Paper 19 and have varying degrees of training offered to midwives (Ward and Spence, 2002; Wright, 2003) but again with limited, or an absence of, evidence from the women themselves to inform policymaking.

Mezey *et al* (2003) carried out a study using focus groups and semi-structured interviews to examine midwives' perceptions and experiences of routine enquiry for domestic violence. The sample of twenty-eight midwives was obtained from the original study which had recruited one hundred and sixteen out of one hundred and forty-five (80%) midwives who were trained to use the abuse assessment screening tool in pregnancy at booking in, thirty-four weeks gestation and postpartum. Results from the twenty-eight midwives found that although the midwives felt that domestic violence was an important issue to be addressed, the midwives encountered practical and personal issues during the study which led the authors to conclude that routine enquiry can only be implemented effectively where there is in-depth training, staff support and adequate resources. Screening was found to be time-consuming, it required skill and experience on the part of the midwife if it was to be helpful to the woman, with an understanding of the midwife's own limitations and responsibility to enable the woman to access appropriate community resources. During the study the authors commented that there was evidence of a raised awareness of the impact domestic abuse has on women's lives and its health consequences, but it was noted that after the study had been completed, virtually all the midwives ceased to ask women about domestic violence. Most of the midwives felt that they needed a specialist midwife who could deal with all the issues relating to domestic violence, including offering them support and a referral system for distressed women. It could be argued that this would take the responsibility away from the midwife who could refer the woman on to the 'domestic violence midwife', with the danger of reinforcing the stigmatisation of domestic violence making it a separate issue from the woman's health, rather than one aspect of a health consultation with a midwife. Midwives are responsible for the majority of, if not all, the care women receive during their childbirth experience. With the emphasis on team working it is hoped that the woman will see the same midwife for either all or for most of her care. This affords the opportunity and potential for a relationship to develop between the woman and her midwife, who has a statutory responsibility to provide care through the childbirth continuum including the postnatal period (Nursing and Midwifer Council [NMC], 2004: 36). Therefore, does enquiry for domestic violence fall inside or outside the role of the midwife? It could be argued that, in accordance with the definition of a midwife (NMC, 2004: 36), it does fall within the responsibilities of the midwife, yet midwives are saying that they are not prepared for this aspect of their role in the form of education or clinical support and would prefer it if others took the responsibility for addressing domestic violence. This consistent response is reflected in those studies cited where midwives have had no training in this area and in those studies where they have had some training.

Disclosure

Disclosure of domestic abuse is an unexplored concept with the debate in health centering on whether to enquire or not. Policy makes the assumption that those women who are experiencing domestic violence, if asked, will be able to disclose within a midwifery encounter. It is well-documented in counselling literature that for a person in a vulnerable state to disclose something personal about themselves, there needs to be a relationship that affords trust, safety and confidentiality. A person-centred approach developed from humanistic theory by Carl Rogers (1951), advocates that the counsellor must display three core conditions to the client, namely; unconditional positive regard, congruence and empathy to enable the client to access his or her phenomenological world. It is questionable as to whether this kind of relationship can be achieved between the woman and her midwife which would facilitate disclosure of domestic abuse. Furthermore, there is limited evidence about the effects on therapists working with people experiencing domestic violence. This area needs to be addressed if midwives are to be placed in the position of actively listening to accounts of physical and emotional cruelty, as not only is it essential that the women receive appropriate and empathic support, but also the midwives themselves. Counsellors are obligated to receive supervision for their counselling practice on a regular basis to ensure that they are working ethically and effectively and also feel supported in their work. There is no such model of supervision in midwifery and there is also limited, and in the main, no support for midwives from their employers should they themselves be experiencing domestic abuse (Trade Union Congress, 2002).

Conclusion

Domestic abuse presents many challenges to midwives in the maternity services. Despite the current debate in the literature regarding routine enquiry, it is evident that domestic abuse is a serious criminal, social and medical problem that has major consequences on the health of many women and children. Statistically it affects one in four women in their lifetime, which means that it is not just the women using the maternity services but the midwives themselves who will have experienced, or will be experiencing domestic abuse.

Policy is dictating that midwives have a responsibility to ask women when they access the maternity services if they are experiencing domestic abuse. Currently, there is limited evidence which says routine enquiry by midwives is effective and will have a positive effect on women's lives and health. In fact, it may have a negative effect if women feel coerced by midwives to leave an abusive relationship without careful and safe planning which could have fatal consequences for the woman and/or her children.

Policy advocates training for midwives and there is an assumption that if training is provided then the training must work and will be incorporated by those trained into their clinical practice. Whilst training midwives was effective for a research study, once the study had been completed the midwives no longer inquired about domestic abuse. It may be more effective to incorporate education about domestic abuse and its impact on health into pre-registration curricula, including the use of effective communication and counselling skills, as part of a life-long learning concept. Other ways of addressing the lack of health professionals knowledge would be the provision of a domestic abuse module to bring current practitioners up-to-date and be educationally informed, thus increasing their confidence to assist women and sign post them to appropriate community resources.

Employers need to support midwives from a two-fold perspective: firstly, supporting midwives to incorporate domestic abuse into their role by providing effective educational opportunities and support/supervision in clinical practice; and secondly from a human resource perspective by supporting midwives who are experiencing domestic abuse themselves. Appointing a domestic abuse coordinator may also help midwives to tackle domestic abuse. A designated person with lead responsibility for domestic abuse would not only raise its profile and visibility in the maternity services, but could input on training and provide support to midwives clinically as well as offering liaison with the professionals and agencies in the community. This model has worked effectively for child protection and could be adapted and adopted locally and nationally for domestic abuse in health. We need to remember that women have limited space of their own in the maternity services. Health professionals in the last twenty to thirty years have actively encouraged partners to accompany women during their pregnancy and birth experience, resulting in an assumption that the partner should always be part of the consultation. For some women this is most acceptable, however, for those women in an abusive relationship it means that they are not afforded the opportunity of a confidential consultation or the opportunity to develop a trusting relationship with the midwife. A practical solution to this problem would be to ensure that at least one antenatal consultation is for the woman on her own, incorporating this into the routine antenatal care guidelines for the maternity services. As midwives we need to be informed of the challenges working with women who experience domestic abuse presents, in order to be able to incorporate routine enquiry into clinical practice to offer effective, empathic and safe care. Working in partnership with the woman will help to empower her and to make choices appropriate for her individual circumstances.

References

Bacchus L, Bewley S, Mezey G (2001) Domestic violence and pregnancy. *Obs Gynae* **3**(2): 56–9

Bacchus L, Mezey G, Bewley S (2002) Women's perceptions and experiences of routine enquiry for domestic violence in a maternity service. *Br J Obstet Gynaecol* **109**: 9–16

Bacchus L, Mezey G, Bewley S (2003) Experiences of seeking help from health professionals in a sample of women who experienced domestic violence. *Health Social Care in the Community* **11**(1): 10–18

Bewley S, Friend J, Mezey G (eds) (1997) *Violence against Women*. RCOG Press, London

Bohn D (1990) Domestic violence and pregnancy implications for practice. *J Nurs Midwifery* **35**(2): 86–8

Bradley F, Smith M, Long J, O'Dowd T (2002) Reported frequency of domestic violence: cross sectional survey of women attending general practice. *Br Med J* **324**: 271–4

British Medical Association (1998) *Domestic Violence: a health care issue?* BMA, London

Brown JB, Lent B, Sas G (1993) Identifying and treating wife abuse. *J Fam Pract* **36**: 185–91

Bullock L, Mc Farlane J, Bateman L H, Miller V (1989) The prevalence and characteristics of battered women in a primary care setting. *Nurse Practitioner* **14**: 47–56

Butler MJ (1995) Domestic violence: a nursing inperative. *J Holistic Nurs* **13**(1): 54–69

Campbell JC, Poland ML, Waller JB, Ager J (1992) Correlates of battering during pregnancy. *Res Nurs Health* **15**: 219–26

Caralis PV, Musialowski R (1997) Women's experiences with domestic violence and their attitudes and expectations regarding medical care of abuse victims. *South Med J* **90**: 1075–80

Confidential Enquiry into Maternal Deaths (2001) *Why Mothers Die 1997–1999. The fifth report of the Confidential Enquiry into Maternal Deaths in the United Kingdom.* RCOG Press, London

Crown Prosecution Service Inspectorate (1998) The Inspectorate's Report on cases involving domestic violence. Thematic Report 2/98. CPS, London

Davison J (1997) Domestic violence: the nursing response. *Prof Nurse* **12**(9): 632–4

Denham S (1995) Confronting the monster of family violence. *Nursing Forum* **30**(3): 12–19

Department of Health (1997) On the state of the Public Health: the Annual Report of the Chief Medical Officer of the Department of Health for the Year 1996. HMSO, London

Department of Health (2000) *Domestic Violence: A resource manual for health care professionals.* DOH, London

Dobash RE, Dobash RP (1979) *Violence against Wives.* Open Books, Shepton Mallett

Dobash RE, Dobash RP, Cavanagh K, Lewis R (1996) *Research evaluation of programmes for violent men.* HMSO, Edinburgh

General Assembly Resolution (1993) The United Nations Declaration on the Elimination of Violence against Women, General Assembly Resolution 48/104 of 20 December 1993

Gilchrist E, Johnson R, Takriti R, Weston S, Beech A, Kebbell M (2003) Domestic violence offenders: characteristics and offending related needs. Home Office Research Study No 217. Home Office, London

Hedin LW (2000) Postpartum, also a risk period for domestic violence. *Eur J Obstet Gynecol Reprod Biol* **89**(1): 41–5

Hillard PJ, (1985) Physical abuse in pregnancy. *Obstet Gynecol* **66**: 185–90

Home Affairs Committee (1993) *Home Affairs Committee Report on Domestic Violence*. HMSO, London

Home Office (1999) *Domestic Violence: findings from a new British Crime Survey self-completion questionnaire*. Home Office Research Studies, London

Hunt SC, Martin AM (2001) *Pregnant Women, Violent Men: What midwives need to know*. Books for Midwives, Oxford

Kershaw C (2000) The 2000 British Crime Survey England and Wales home Office Statistical Bulletin 18/00. Home Office, London

Lovenduski J, Randall V (1993) *Contemporary Feminist Politics: Women and Power*. Oxford University Press, London

McFarlane J, Parker B, Soeken K (1996) Physical abuse, smoking and substance use during pregnancy: prevalence, interrelationships and effects on birth weight. *J Obstet Gynecol Neonatal Nurs* **25**: 313–20

McFarlane J, Parker B, Soeken K, Bullock L (1992) Assessing for abuse during pregnancy: severity and frequency of injuries and associated entry into prenatal care. *JAMA* **267**: 3176–8

Marchant S, Davidson LL, Garcia J, Parsons JE (2001) Addressing domestic violence through maternity services: policy and practice. *Midwifery* **17**:164–70

Mayhew P, Mirlees-Black C, Percy A (1996) The 1996 British Crime Survey England and Wales. Home Office Statistical Bulletin, Issue 19/96. Home Office, London

Mezey GC (1997) Domestic violence and pregnancy. In: Bewley S, Friend J, Mezey G, eds. *Violence against Women*. RCOG Press, London

Mezey GC, Bewley S (1997) Domestic violence and pregnancy. *Br J Obstet Gynecol* **104**: 528–31

Mezey G, Bachus L, Haworth A, Bewley S (2003) Midwives' perceptions and experiences of routine enquiry for domestic violence. *Br J Obstet Gynaecol* **110**: 744–52

Miller MS (1995) *No Visible Wounds: Identifying non-physical abuse of women by their men*. Fawcett Columbine, New York

Mirrlees-Black C, Byron C (1999) *Domestic Violence: Findings from the BCS self-completion questionnaire*. Research Findings No 86, Home Office Research, Development and Statistics Directorate. Home Office, London

Mooney J (1993) *The Hidden Figure: Domestic violence in north London*. Islington Council, London

Morgan JE (2003) Knowledge and experience of domestic violence. *Br J Midwifery* **12**(11): 741–7

NHS Executive ((1998) Confidential enquiries into maternal deaths 1994–1996. Wetherby: HSC 1998/211

National Institute for Clinical Excellence (2003) *Antenatal Care. Routine care for the healthy pregnant woman*. Clinical Guideline 6. NICE, London

Nursing and Midwifery Council (2004) *Midwives Rules and Standards*. NMC, London

O'Campo P, Gielen AC, Faden RR, Kass N (1994) Verbal abuse and physical violence among a cohort of low-income pregnant women. *Women's Health Issues* **4**: 29–37

Peckover S (2001) *Professional Briefing, Domestic Violence: A framework of good practice.* The Community Practitioners' and Health Visitors' Association (CPHVA), London

Ramsay J, Richardson J, Carter YH, Davidson LL, Feder G (2002) Should health professionals screen women for domestic violence? Systematic review. *Br Med J* **325**: 314–8

Ramsay J, Richardson J, Carter YH, Davidson LL, Feder G (2002) Letters, Safe. *Domestic Abuse Quarterly* **3**:20

Richardson J, Feder G (1996) Domestic violence: a hidden problem for general practice. *Br J Gen Prac* April: 239–42

Richardson J, Coid J, Petruckevitch A, Chung W S, Moorey S, Feder G (2002) Identifying domestic violence: cross-sectional study in primary care. *Br Med J* **324**: 274–7

Rogers C (1951) *Client-centred Therapy: its current practice, implications and theory.* Houghton Mifflin, Boston

Royal College of Midwives (1997) *Domestic Abuse in Pregnancy.* RCM Position Paper No 19. RCM, Cardiff

Royal College of Nursing (2000) *Domestic Violence. Guidance for Nurses.* RCN, London

Sampselle CM, Peterson BA, Murtland TL, Oakley DJ (1992) Prevalence of abuse among pregnant women choosing certified nurse-midwife or physician providers. *J Nurs Midwifery* **37**: 269–73

Schornstein SL (1997) *Domestic Violence and Healthcare. What every professional needs to know.* Sage, London

Scobie J, McGuire M (1999) The silent enemy: domestic violence in pregnancy. *Br J Midwif* **7**(4): 259–62

Secretary of State for Health (1997) *The New NHS: modern dependable.* CM 3807

Shumway J, O'Campo P, Gielen A, Witter FR, Khouzami AN, Blakemore KJ (1999) Preterm labour, placental abruption and premature rupture of membranes in relation to maternal violence or verbal abuse. *J Mat Fet Med* **179**: 76-80

Stanko E, Crisp D, Hale C, Lutcraft H (1997) Counting the costs: estimating the impact of domestic violence in the London Borough of Hackney. In: British Medical Association (1998) (ed) *Domestic Violence: a health care issue?* BMA, London

Stark E, Flitcraft A (1996) *Women at Risk: Domestic violence and women's health.* Sage, London

Stenson K, Saarinen H, Heimer G, Sidenvall B (2001) Women's attitudes to being asked about exposure to violence. *Midwifery* **17**: 2–10

Stewart DE, Cecutti A (1993) Physical abuse in pregnancy. *Can Med Assoc J* **149**: 1257-63

Sugg N K, Inui T (1992) Primary care physicians' response to domestic violence. Opening Pandora's Box. *JAMA* **267**(23): 3157–60

Taket A, Nurse J, Smith K, Watson J, Shakespeare J, Lavis V, Cosgrove K, Mulley K, Feder G (2003) Routinely asking women about domestic violence in healthcare settings. *Br Med J* **327**: 673–6

Trade Union Congress (2002) *Domestic violence: A guide for the workplace.* TUC, London
UNICEF (2000) *Domestic Violence Against Women and Girls.* No 6, June. UNICEF Innocenti Research Centre, Italy
Walker L (1984) *The Battered Women's Syndrome.* Springer, New York
Ward S, Spence A (2002) Training midwives to screen for domestic violence. MIDIRS *Midwifery Digest* **12**(1): S15–S17
Webster J, Stratigos SM, Grimes KM (2001) Women's responses to screening for domestic violence in a health-care setting. *Midwifery* **17**: 289–94
Williamson E (2000) *Domestic violence and health. The response of the medical profession.* Policy Press, Bristol
World Health Organization (2002) *World Report on Violence and Health.* WHO, Geneva
World Medical Association (1996) Declaration on family violence. Adopted by the 48th General Assembly, October, 1996, South Africa
Wright L (2003) Asking about domestic violence. *Br J Midwifery* **11**(4): 199–202

9

Assessing the quality of maternity care for Pakistani and indigenous 'white' women

Janet Hirst and Jenny Hewison

Assessing the quality of maternity care is not new. Since the 1930s the providers of the maternity services have evaluated outcomes, in terms of maternal and perinatal mortality, as an indicator of its effectiveness. Initially it was assumed that general improvements in the maternal and perinatal mortality rates (particularly since the introduction of the National Health Service) were directly related to technological advances in maternity care and the shift of care from the community to the hospital (Macfarlane and Mugford, 1984). However, a contemporary view is that improvements in both maternal and perinatal mortality rates are reflective of a much broader social picture, which include improvements to women's lifestyles, health, education, and standards of living, as well as changes to the content and frequency of maternity care (Tew, 1990). These views are more realistic and are partly supported by the fact that such improvements have changed at different rates for different groups of women and that they have been inextricably linked to women's lifestyles, general health, education and standards of living (Townsend and Davidson, 1982; Whitehead, 1987; Ahmad, 1989; Balarajan and Raleigh, 1993; Confidential Enquiry into Maternal Deaths, 2001; House of Commons, 2003a; Richens, 2003).

It is wrong to assume that everyone wants or needs the same content of maternity care. Social, cultural and religious obligations, for example, may affect choices that women make about the process of their maternity care; such as their preference for the type of care giver or the gender of that carer. It is also wrong to assume that equity is about providing women with the same choices, as such choices may be irrelevant and irrelevance is a poor indicator of service quality (Maxwell 1992; Schott and Henley, 1996: 48; Hirst and Hewison, 2001).

We know that the way in which women from different backgrounds use the maternity services and the way in which the service is provided for women differ. What is unclear is whether such differences affect the quality of service as perceived by women. In this context, quality refers to users' views of the process of care; ie. what was delivered, by whom and in what way, such as the technical care received, the interpersonal experience that took place and the circumstances in which care took place. Achieving 'high quality' care is an aspiration of NHS organisations and strategies are in place to enable this, ie. the system of clinical governance. Currently, an aspect of quality receiving particular attention is the way in which women access maternity care (House of Commons, 2003a). There is evidence to show that how care is perceived and how satisfied women are depends on what women wanted from the service; and it is clear that what women want and expect influences their satisfaction with care (Green *et al*, 1990). It has also been indicated that a strong internal locus of control may modulate negative experiences (Spirito *et al*, 1990), ie. the extent to which women believe they can influence their own health and that women's experience and views of their pregnancy are affected by whom women believe control the outcome of pregnancy (Tinsley *et al*, 1993).

Measuring satisfaction has been highlighted as an important factor in the assessment of quality. The complexity of associating women's satisfaction with their maternity care can be illustrated as follows. It has been found that women's preferences tend to be shaped by what was available, and that women have tended to like what they have experienced (Porter and McIntyre, 1984). However, one must be cautious at drawing any assumption that 'women like what they get', as other studies have shown that although most women report that they like the care they have received, the proportion of women who report this varies and this variation is associated with the type of carer (Hill *et al*, 1993; Hirst *et al*, 1996, Hirst *et al*, 1998). Therefore, the association between the provision of care and women's satisfaction with care is more dynamic than Porter and McIntyre suggest.

It has been considered that the extent to which users are satisfied with their health care is associated with their expectations, and that expectations can be modified through the process of care (Donabedian, 1992; Williams, 1994). Potentially, if users' expectations are raised the quality of the service would need to meet such expectations to maintain a high satisfaction rating. However, one could argue that it is not in the interest of managers of health care to raise users' expectations above and beyond what can be realistically delivered, or above and beyond what is clinically effective; and it is not in the interest of the users of the service to have their expectations raised above what they are likely to get, as Green *et al* (1990) have shown.

A number of theorists have attempted to model the relationship between users' expectations, preferences and satisfaction of healthcare (Williams, 1994); yet the relationships remain complex and unclear and without any consensus of opinion (Williams, 1994; Martin-Hirsch and Wright, 1998). An explanation for this is that users' expectations and preferences are determined by other factors such as previous experiences, the type of information that is given, and personal and social characteristics (Green *et al*, 1990; Williams, 1994; Rudat *et al*, 1993; Martin-Hirsch and Wright, 1998). Therefore, those that have used and developed user rated satisfaction scales have not overcome the fundamental problem that global satisfaction ratings of health care are thought to be of little value. In addition, specific ratings need to be interpreted with caution, as there is no consensus that what is being measured is directly related to the service, or that users actually express their true feelings. The consensus is that user rated satisfaction scales are problematic and recent evaluations of healthcare services, particularly in maternity care, are moving away from such problematic measurements towards qualitative methods.

Some surveys that have used qualitative approaches to obtain women's views about care analysed qualitative data in such a way that women's positive and negative comments were reported for each phase of maternity care and used as an indicator of women's perceptions of the quality of care (Garcia *et al*, 1998; Proctor and Wright, 1998; Hirst *et al*, 1998). A value of presenting women's views in this way is that it shows where phases of maternity services are meeting or failing the needs of women. By obtaining women's views of their care, Proctor and Wright (1998) point out that women comment upon aspects that either 'impress' or 'bother' them in some way. They also report that there may be no relationship between these 'impressions' and women's initial preferences for care or expectations of care.

Having established that assessing women's views of satisfaction has pitfalls, we can also show that women's pregnancy-related locus of control may influence women's views of care. For example, there is evidence to support the view that people who have a high internal locus of control (that is the extent to which people believe that personal behaviour can influence their health) assume more responsibility for their health, guard against accidents and disease, seek more information about health maintenance and learn more about their illness (Tinsley *et al*, 1993). Such women may have different requirements from the service than women with high external locus of control (ie. those who assume that healthcare professionals and the play of chance have a greater influence upon their health than their own actions). It is also conceivable that religion influences 'who' women regard as responsible for the health of their un-born baby. Tinsley *et al* (1993) have reported that pregnancy-related locus of control beliefs appear to contribute to individual differences in women's antenatal health behaviour and birth outcome. Surveys that have obtained the views of women, as a measure of the quality of their maternity care, have shown that women's views differ. The reasons why they differ are reported to be due to a number of factors; such as, women's preferences, expectations, psychological well-being, ethnicity, culture, language, religion, family support, socio-economic status, the experience of care and women's personality traits, eg. locus of control (Green *et al*, 1990; Bielawska-Batorowicz, 1993; Tinsley *et al*, 1993; Rudat, 1993; Quine *et al*, 1993; Ogden *et al*, 1998; Garcia *et al*, 1998; Martin-Hirsch and Wright, 1998; Hirst and Hewison, 2002). With regard to pregnancy and childbirth the Fetal Health Locus of Control Scale (FHLC) (Labs and Wurtele, 1986) has been designed and validated to measure a woman's locus of control specifically related to the health of her un-born baby and her health-related behaviour during pregnancy. Subsequently, it has been suggested that a woman's pregnancy-related locus of control could influence their view of care and carers (Bielawska-Batorowicz, 1993; Tinsley *et al*, 1993). Therefore, assessing women's pregnancy-related locus of control may be useful in explaining and understanding women's views of care and such data for Pakistani and indigenous 'white' women will be presented in this chapter.

There is a clear message within the literature that the views of women are important indicators of the quality of the maternity services. In addition, it is clear that the views of some women have been insufficiently captured or captured in such a way that their views are not heard, ie. their views are overwhelmed by a majority consensus (DoH, 1993; Bowes and Domokos, 1996; House of Commons, 2003a). This chapter offers insight into data that were collected during 1994 and 1995 relating to women's preferences for and views of antenatal care, in particular, place of care and the type of carer; and whilst this seems some time ago the results and issues are still pertinent for contemporary maternity services (House of Commons, 2003a; House of Commons, 2003b). The data were drawn from a study that set out to obtain the views of Pakistani and indigenous 'white' women as a means to assess their preferences and views of the quality of maternity care (Hirst, 1999). This chapter considers data regarding antenatal care and women's pregnancy-related locus of control.

Methods

The study was a prospective comparative survey and women were recruited to the study from health centres in two health districts in the north of England between July 1995 and August 1996. As with many studies underpinned by a qualitative approach, the sample size was based upon pragmatic reasoning (Mays and Pope, 1996: 34). For this study, sufficient numbers of women were required so that the data could be compared, a manageable amount of qualitative data analysed and new insights gained. Another consideration was that although the recruitment rate was anticipated to be good, as shown by other studies (Rudat *et al*, 1993), the number of women who would agree to the second interview could not be predicted. The target number of participants was therefore 100 (fifty Pakistani women and fifty indigenous 'white' women), to allow for attrition the target recruitment number was 152 (seventy-six Pakistani women and seventy-six indigenous 'white' women). Generalisability was not the most important feature of the sampling process; obtaining a sample of appropriate women was the main intention and this underpins the appropriateness of using non-probability sampling techniques, ie. purposive sampling (Field and Morse, 1992: 95; Moser and Kalton, 1996: 82). The views of women were obtained using qualitative tools, by way of two face-to-face interviews, using a semi-structured schedule for the antenatal interview and an in-depth interview schedule for the postnatal interview. An aim of the antenatal interview was to collect data around the pattern and frequency of maternity care as well as women's views (preferences and expectations) of their care; hence a semi-structured schedule was an obvious choice. An aim of the postnatal interview was particularly to allow women to disclose issues that were important to them;

therefore, a more open and in-depth approach was considered to be appropriate. All interviews took place in the participant's home, recorded by handwritten notes and checked for validity at the time of the interview. The first interview took place before the participants were thirty weeks pregnant and the second between six and eight weeks after the birth; each interview lasted about one hour. In addition, data were collected from maternity casenotes for all women who undertook the first interview using a pre-planned proforma to document the pattern of care. A bilingual researcher assisted with the recruitment and interviewing of women who did not understand or speak English very well. The interviews yielded a vast amount of qualitative data that were analysed using a content analysis technique (Burnard, 1991; Field and Morse, 1992) and a sample of data coding was informally checked for quality between two independent researchers. Overall, there was a high degree of agreement and where inconsistencies occurred these were resolved through discussion. The frequencies of data were treated as nominal levels of measurement; cross tabulations and chi square test for association were used where appropriate. Other quantitative analysis included analysis of variance for unmatched groups (ANOVA) for ratio data, eg. the gestation of pregnancy. The following results were compared between ethnic groups and or districts as a means to assess whether differences could be associated with ethnicity or with a district.

Two hundred and twenty-five women were asked to take part in the study, 187 (83%) agreed. Of these, 153 took part with the first interview (68% of the total asked: seventy-six were Pakistani and seventy-seven indigenous 'white' women) and of the 143 women eligible for the second interview, 139 (97%) took part. The main language of the Pakistani women in both districts was Punjabi and fifty Pakistani women requested an interpreter as they did not speak English very well, or at all (100 interviews interpreted). Grouping women from different ethnic groups into social classifications was problematic as families from different ethnic groups used financial resources differently; hence, this characteristic had little value and has been omitted. There were highly significant differences between the ethnic groups regarding the level of education that women achieved as most of the Pakistani women did not have any formal qualifications. Other differences were that more of the indigenous 'white' women were having their first pregnancy; only five of the Pakistani women were employed, either full or part-time, compared to forty-six indigenous 'white' women; and more of the Pakistani women were under twenty years of age.

Early pregnancy

The gestation of pregnancy when women present for the first antenatal visit (often called a booking visit), the health professional that women see and the venue have been topics of debate for some time. However, to be able to understand these issues we need to have insight into when women first knew that they were pregnant and when pregnancy was confirmed. For these women the mean gestation when they first thought they were pregnant was 6.4 weeks (sd 2.9) and the mean gestation for the confirmation of pregnancy 8 weeks (sd 3.5). The differences between districts (A and B) and between ethnic groups were statistically significant, however, all women had their pregnancy confirmed during the first trimester, which was desirable (F=13.0, df=1, 144, P<.001 and F=6.9, df=1, 144, P=.009 respectively). Indigenous 'white' women in district A knew that they were pregnant and confirmed their pregnancy much earlier than the other women; subsequently, these women received their first antenatal visit earlier.

Table 9.1: The gestation when women first thought that they were pregnant				
(Mean number of weeks)	District A: Indigenous 'white' women	District A: Pakistani women	District B: Indigenous 'white' women	District B: Pakistani women
Gestation when first thought pregnant	4.8	6.2	7.0	7.8
Mean gesta-tion when pregnancy confirmed*	5.8	8.4	8.9	9.1
(F*=13.0, df=1, 144, P<.001 and F=6.9, df=1, 144, P=0.009)				

Ensuring that women are offered choices regarding maternity care is an important quality indicator for service providers and highly profiled by *Changing Childbirth* (DoH, 1993) and subsequent reports (House of Commons, 2003b). Out of 146 women in this study, 76% (n 111) perceived that they had a choice about who they could see and 72% (n 105) perceived that they had a choice about where they could go to have their pregnancy confirmed. Twenty-four percent of women (n 35) did not perceive that they had a choice about who they could see (twenty-nine were Pakistani) and 29% (n 42) did not perceive that they had a choice about where they could go, again most were Pakistani (n 35), to confirm their pregnancy. Of course, we cannot assume that all of these women wanted such choices and, indeed, they did not as fourteen women (thirteen Pakistani) out of thirty-five wanted more information about who they could see to confirm their pregnancy and nineteen women (eighteen Pakistani) out of forty-two wanted more information about where they could go.

Women were asked who they would like to see to confirm their pregnancy out of a list of options. Overall, 40% (n 60) of women preferred a general practitioner. However, thirty-three of the seventy-six indigenous 'white' women commented that they preferred to do the pregnancy test themselves at home, whereas Pakistani women commented on a range of options (*Table 9.2*).

The most frequently reported reason why women held a preference for a particular 'carer' to confirm their pregnancy was as a means to access an accurate test and a speedy result; this was mainly within the indigenous 'white' group. The most frequent comments made by Pakistani women referred to gender of the carer, perceived technical competency of the carer and ambivalence, 'I just wanted to know'. Patterns emerged within some practices where Pakistani women received the result of their pregnancy test from a female member of the administrative staff (GP receptionist); for some women this was unacceptable even though she was a woman, as she lacked technical competence.

Table 9.2: Women's preferred carer for the confirmation of pregnancy

	Indigenous 'white' women	Pakistani women	Total (%) n=150
GP	26	34	60 (40%)
Self-testing	33	3	36 (24%)
Midwife	0	13	13 (9%)
Pharmacist	9	4	13 (9%)
Anyone	0	12	12 (8%)
GP receptionist	1	4	5 (3%)
Practice nurse, family planning clinic	3	1	4 (3%)
Other, ie. drop-in centres	4	3	7 (5%)

In summary, both Pakistani and indigenous 'white' women confirmed their pregnancy during the first trimester of pregnancy, which is a similar finding to other authors (Shiekh and Theodore-Ghandi, 1988; Rudat *et al*, 1993; Garcia *et al*, 1998) and most women, in both ethnic groups, reported that they had a choice about whom they could see and where they could go to have their pregnancy confirmed; those who did not were likely to be Pakistani women. Different ethnic groups favoured confirming their pregnancy in different ways, accuracy and speed of the result and the gender of the carer being important components that could influence new and innovative ways to offer early antenatal care.

The first antenatal visit

The first antenatal visit (the booking visit) is a significant event for many women as they often commence new relationships with carers, become familiar with a plethora of information and make personal health-related decisions and health-related choices for their unborn baby; particularly in relation to prenatal screening. Currently, the desired gestation for the first antenatal visit is prior to twelve weeks (NICE, 2003). The mean gestation for the first antenatal visit for all women in this study was 10.7 weeks (sd 3.9), indigenous 'white' women in district A were the earliest at 8.7 weeks and Pakistani women in district B the latest at 12 weeks. The differences between the district and ethnic groups reflected the same patterns as for when women first thought that they were pregnant and when they had their pregnancy confirmed.

Most women (124, 81%) saw the midwife at this first visit, there were no differences between the districts, ethnic groups or within the districts. The remaining women saw the GP (thirteen), combination of carers (ten) or the obstetrician (seven). Of the seventy-six Pakistani women, sixteen reported that they also saw a linkworker (linkworkers provided interpreting services between carers and users in the hospital and community settings in both districts), fifteen of these women were in district B (in district A Pakistani women had access to a community midwife who was fluent in their own language). The place of the first antenatal visit for nearly all women (130, 86%) was at the GP surgery/health centre. There were no significant differences between the district or ethnic groups for this pattern. Overall, most women perceived that they had no choice about who they could see for their first antenatal visit or where it could have taken place. Of the 116 women who reported that they had no choice about whom they could see, only twenty-eight said that they would have liked a choice; these were mainly Pakistani (twenty-one) and mainly from district A (twelve).

Most women (119) did not know that they had a choice about where they could be seen for their first antenatal visit. On this occasion, Pakistani women were more likely to comment that they had a choice and indigenous 'white' women more likely to report that they did not. Within district B, this difference was statistically significant ($x2$ =7.0, df−1, P=.008). Of the 119 women who reported that they had no choice, forty would have liked a choice and these women were equally distributed between the districts; however, more of the Pakistani women would have liked a choice compared to indigenous 'white' women ($x2$ = 14.11, df=1. P<.001).

Overall, women preferred to see the midwife at their first antenatal visit, which was what most women received. However, there were significant differences between the ethnic groups regarding who women preferred to see. Pakistani women were more likely to prefer their GP and other combinations of carers than the midwife on her own than indigenous 'white' women ($x2$ = 12.7, df=3, P=.005). *Table 9.3* shows who women would like to see for their first antenatal visit.

Women's preference for their carer was found to be more complex than simply choosing a professional type as most preferences were underpinned by conditional characteristics of carers and worded in such a way as to indicate that they were a prerequisite; the term '... as long as' usually being used to indicate this. In 62% (n 95) of the first interviews (n 153), women gave up to two un-prompted responses regarding their preference for antenatal carers. The conditional characteristics that women gave most frequently related to gender of carer, ie. '... as long as she is a woman' and continuity, ie. '... as long as it's one from the team'. A comparison between the number of women who mentioned only gender compared to those who mentioned continuity or gender and continuity was found to be statistically significant between the districts ($x2 = 21.6$, df=2, P<.001) and between the ethnic groups ($x2=20.3$, df=2, P<.001). The most important condition 'gender' of the carer was mainly, but not exclusively, reported by Pakistani women particularly in district B; in district A continuity featured more frequently.

Table 9.3: The carer whom women preferred to see for their first antenatal visit

	Indigenous 'white' women	Pakistani women	Total (%) n=151
Midwife	53	39	92 (61%)
GP	9	15	24 (16%)
Midwife or GP or obstetrician	3	14	17 (11%)
Other combinations of these carers	12	6	18 (12%)
2 missing observations (Between the ethnic groups χ^2=12.7, df=3, P=.005)			

Table 9.4: The conditions women gave regarding their choice of carer for their first antenatal visit

	Indigenous 'white' women	Pakistani women	Total (%) n=90
Gender	15	40	55 (61%)
Continuity	14	7	21 (23%)
Gender and continuity	12	2	14 (16%)
(Between the districts χ^2=21.6, df=2, P<.001 and between the ethnic groups χ^2=20.3, df=2, P<.001)			

The reasons why women held a preference for a particular carer (for the first antenatal visit) were explored and 143 women gave up to three reasons. Content analysis of these data revealed three main themes: perceived roles and technical competency, gender of carer and continuity. Perceived roles and technical competency of carer were mentioned by 51% (n 73) of women, the main reasons being that '...the midwife is a specialist' or '...it's her (the midwife's) job'. Gender of carer was mentioned by 40% (n 65) of women, mostly Pakistani, ie. '...because she is a woman', and continuity by 17% (n 24) of women, mainly in district A, eg. '...you get to know them well'. The data were analysed further and compared regarding the number of women who mentioned gender and those who did not. It was found to be statistically significant in that Pakistani women mentioned it most frequently (χ^2=20.1, df=1, P<.001).

In summary, in relation to the first antenatal visit significant differences were found between ethnic groups. In particular, more of the Pakistani women preferred the general practitioner or combinations of carers (including the midwife), as long as they were female. Indigenous 'white' women were more likely to comment upon aspects of continuity, in particular continuity of a carer; and it was significant that the Pakistani women in district B perceived that they had no choice around where they could be seen for their first visit. Whilst other authors have reported that women 'like what they get' (Porter and McIntyre, 1984), this research adds to the knowledge that this is not always the case (Hirst *et al*, 1996). In addition, where women did not perceive to have a choice, Pakistani women were more likely to want one. From these data it was clear that women preferred flexibility in service provision which appear fairly easy to provide but less easy to manage, monitor and ensure that all carers continue with appropriate professional development.

Subsequent antenatal care

The pattern, frequency and effectiveness of antenatal care have been under scrutiny for some time and has more recently been a focus for the National Institute for Clinical Excellence (NICE, 2003). Contemporary guidelines have identified the optimum pattern and frequency of antenatal care where neither the health of the woman or fetus are compromised. For the 114 women (where full data were available) in this study the mean number of antenatal visits for all groups was 12.8 (sd 3.1), which is slightly more than (>1-2) contemporary guidelines recommend; indigenous 'white' women in both districts having two antenatal visits more than Pakistani women. Most antenatal care took place at the GP surgery/health centre and the mean number of community antenatal visits was 9.9 (sd = 4). All women in district B attended the hospital more frequently than in district A but this did not reach statistical significance. Different trends in the patterns of subsequent antenatal visits, between the ethnic groups, could be explained because more of the indigenous 'white' women knew that they were pregnant earlier and began their maternity care sooner than Pakistani women. Another factor was that more of the indigenous 'white' women were having their first pregnancy.

It was not clear from the maternity records which carer women saw at each antenatal visit as practitioners signed their name but rarely wrote their designation. Such data were, therefore, unreliable and not reported. However, the number of different signatures of carers for each antenatal visit was thought to be a reasonable indicator of continuity of carer. In the community setting, differences occurred between ethnic groups, and in the hospital setting between the districts. A comparison of the mean number of signatures in the community setting found that Pakistani women were more likely to see a fewer number of carers even though they were less likely to receive care from midwifery 'teams' ($F=25.6$, df=1,87, $P<.001$), and a comparison of the mean number of signatures in the hospital setting found that women in district A were more likely to see fewer carers than district B ($F=29.5$, df=1,105, $P<.001$).

Women were asked which carers they preferred to see for their antenatal care and the midwife and the GP were mentioned most frequently. However, analysis of these data found that some women specifically preferred the midwife or they specifically preferred the GP, other women preferred the midwife and the GP, and some women didn't mind and commented the midwife or the GP. The hospital obstetrician was mentioned by ten women and again these responses included combinations of other carers. As *Table 9.5* shows, it appears that the presence of a midwife was important for most women, but not necessarily on her own, and the role of the GP and the hospital obstetrician played an important part of their maternity care.

Table 9.5: The carer whom women preferred to see for their subsequent antenatal visit			
	Indigenous 'white' women	Pakistani women	Total (%) n=153
Midwife	30	28	58 (38%)
Midwife or GP	14	21	35 (23%)
Midwife or GP or hospital doctor	14	16	30 (20%)
Other combinations of these carers	19	11	30 (20%)

Again, women's preference for their carers was found to be more complex than simply choosing a professional type, as 74% (n 113) of women gave at least one conditional requirement of their choice of carer (up to two conditions were given). There were no significant differences between the districts but there were differences between the ethnic groups in that the gender of carer was mentioned by more of the Pakistani women and continuity by more of the indigenous 'white' women; however, in neither case were these conditions exclusive to one ethnic group. Overall, comments were similar to women's preferences for the first antenatal visit in that the most frequently made comment regarding the gender of carer was '... as long as it's a woman', and 'I prefer a woman' and for continuity, 'I prefer the same one' or 'I prefer one from the team, a regular one'. For fourteen women both gender and continuity were important conditions.

Women were asked why they preferred carers and were able to give at least one reason (some women gave up to three). Women's perception of carers' role and competency was mentioned most often, the main comments being, '...it's the midwives job' or '...it's the GP's job'. For those who liked combinations of carers they said, '... it's best to get everyone involved so that you get different opinions' and those who did not mind commented that, '... they all know as much as each other'. Roles and technical competency were commented upon most frequently by indigenous 'white' women in both districts, whereas the gender of carer was commented more frequently by Pakistani women. Overall, there were 338 positive and 108 negative comments regarding women's carers. *Tables 9.6* and *9.7* show the number of women who made a positive and a negative comment in each of the key themes.

Table 9.6: The positive comments regarding antenatal care

+ve	Indigenous 'white' women	Pakistani women	Total (%) n=139
Continuity	60	47	107 (77%)
Information	24	41	65 (48%)
Technical competency	13	33	46 (33%)
Interpersonal skills	22	11	33 (24%)
Psychological well-being	18	12	30 (22%)
(A woman may have commented in more than one theme)			

Table 9.7: The negative comments regarding antenatal care

-ve	Indigenous 'white' women	Pakistani women	Total (%) n=139
Information	26	9	35 (25%)
Interpersonal skills/ type of carer	14	5	19 (14%)
Technical competency	12	4	16 (12%)
(A woman may have commented in more than one theme)			

It is worth mentioning that coding data within themes was, sometimes, difficult as it was difficult to separate 'continuity' from 'perceived technical skill'. For fifty-nine women not seeing the same carer prompted a positive response, a frequent comment was, '...it didn't really matter seeing different community midwives as they all did the same thing' and for another sixteen women, 'I didn't mind who I saw as long as they did everything right'. For women who did see the same carers seventeen said that they, 'liked' this, however, it is not clear exactly how many carers women saw. Overall, indigenous 'white' women in both districts gave most of the positive comments and there were very few negative comments in this theme.

With regard to information giving, Pakistani women in both districts gave more of the positive comments and indigenous 'white' women in both districts more of the negative comments. Women who gave a positive comment reported receiving information such as, '...how to look after myself' and '...what I should and shouldn't eat'. Negative comments tended to be about women feeling that 'I didn't learn anything new' or 'particularly helpful' or that 'I didn't learn enough'.

The most frequent positive comment about the technical care was that it was 'good' and for forty women this meant that their carers listened, explained everything, checked everything and solved their problems. Most women who made a negative comment said that their care was 'poor'; this meant that carers were not bothered about them and women were not informed about the results of antenatal checks and tests.

Positive comments made most frequently regarding carers' interpersonal skills related to the community midwife. In particular, community midwives were '...all really nice', 'friendly' and '...give the impression that they have time for you'. Of the small number of women who did make a negative comment, seven women wanted to see their consultant obstetrician more because they liked them.

The most frequent positive comments regarding women's psychological well-being were that women felt reassured, confident and comfortable with their carers. A small number of women received care from 'team midwives' and four of these women made comments such as, '... it's nice to think that you will see the one you know when you have your baby'. There were very few negative comments in this theme.

For most women the largest proportion of subsequent antenatal care was held at the GP surgery/health centre. Only half of the women who had a second interview made any comment about this, thirty-eight women made at least one positive comment (up to two comments given) and twenty-six women made at least one negative comment. Positive comments were generally about the ease of getting to the surgery and shorter waiting times (than the hospital), whereas negative comments were mainly about having to wait a long time and the surgery having out-of-date equipment. There were little differences between the district and ethnic groups regarding the proportion of positive and negative comments, although indigenous 'white' women in both places tended to give most of the negative comments.

Only twenty-eight women made any comment about the hospital venue regarding their antenatal care. Twenty women made at least one negative comment (up to two) and these focused around long waiting times and the carers not doing anything different. Although the numbers were small, negative comments were mainly given by women in district B (where women attended the hospital more) and again mainly by indigenous 'white' women. Very few women had any antenatal care at home to report.

Fifty-one women were admitted into hospital at least once during their antenatal period (not antenatal day unit), fifteen of these women were admitted twice and five of these women three times or more. The main reasons for admission were: early onset of labour, prior to an induction of labour, antenatal vaginal bleeding, suspected spontaneous rupture of membranes or other obstetric or medical indications. There were little differences between the district or ethnic groups regarding the number of women who were admitted, however, indigenous 'white' women tended to be admitted more frequently. Women who were admitted gave twenty-eight positive and forty negative comments about their stay. Most of the positive comments referred to women enjoying their stay (ten women) and that the staff '...were nice' (ten women). Sixteen women made a negative comment: mainly that the ward was too noisy, too hot, visiting times too short or too strict. A further thirteen women commented that they were bored, fed up, frightened or worried. There were no significant differences between the districts, however, most of the negative comments were made by indigenous 'white' women.

The small differences between the districts regarding the number of times women attended the hospital for antenatal care could be explained by different ways of organising 'shared care' between the lead carers (the GP and an obstetrician). Analysis of data extracted from the maternity records found that it was significant that Pakistani women, in both districts, were seen by a fewer number of different carers, therefore receiving a better continuity of carer. This was unexpected because the Pakistani women were less likely to be cared for by midwifery teams (midwifery teams operationalisde the concept of continuity of carer and continuity of care as a means to improve the quality of maternity services). However, more of the Pakistani women were registered with a 'single GP practice'.

A comparison of women's preferences regarding their carer found a number of important differences in the trends between ethnic groups. It was evident that the presence of a 'single' midwife for antenatal care was preferred by most women. However, other combinations of carers were acceptable for many as long as 'conditional' requirements were met. It was notable that Pakistani women's preference for a female carer was particularly strong, a finding that has been well documented (Bowes and Domokos, 1996; DoH, 1993; Hemingway *et al*, 1994; Woollett *et al*, 1995). It was also important that a preference for a female carer was mentioned by a number of indigenous 'white' women, particularly in district B. What this study has shown was that there were no homogenous groups regarding preferences for a particular gender of carer, or continuity of carer or women's ability to assess their carers' competency.

The main reason that women preferred particular carers was their perception of their carers' professional roles and competency. In addition to this, many Pakistani women viewed gender and many indigenous 'white' women viewed continuity as important reasons for explaining their preferences. When women reflected upon their antenatal experience, the theme 'continuity' was frequently commented upon by all groups of women. The item within this theme now focused around the positive aspects of seeing a carer that they did not know. On this occasion, this information supports other studies that have shown that women tend to like the care that they receive (Porter and McIntyre, 1984) and, indeed, there were fewer negative than positive comments regarding women's antenatal visits. However, this trend was not apparent for all aspects of antenatal care, as most women who were admitted to the hospital antenatal ward reported a negative experience.

Other authors have reported that Pakistani women are reluctant to complain about their care (Rudat et al, 1993) and despite the interview schedule being developed in such a way as to minimise this, indigenous 'white' women were more likely to express a negative experience. One example of this related to the comments women made about information. Pakistani women made most of the positive comments and indigenous 'white' women most of the negative comments. It could have been that Pakistani women perceived that they had gained new information, particularly about pregnancy and childbirth practices in the UK, whilst indigenous 'white' women did not develop any new knowledge or knowledge that was not easily accessible from other sources.

It was surprising that 'communication' did not emerge as a key theme from the second interview, particularly amongst Pakistani women but also with indigenous 'white' women as communication underpins all aspects of maternity care (Rudat et al, 1993; Green and France-Dawson, 1994; Gready et al, 1995; Schott and Henley, 1996). However, reference to communication did occur but did not emerge as a key theme. This was partly because of the approach to the qualitative analysis and partly because the frequency which women directly referred to communication was small. However, reference to communication indirectly and directly included Pakistani and indigenous 'white' women. For example, a small number of women from both ethnic groups commented that, 'It is easier talking to a woman', which was coded as a positive aspect within the theme of gender. A Pakistani woman reported that, '…you can talk to a doctor about certain things' and an indigenous 'white' woman reported, 'I understand the midwife more, they talk at your level'. Both of these comments were coded positively within the theme of roles and technical competency. In contrast, there were a small number of direct comments relating to communication. In particular, a Pakistani women's preference for carer carried a conditional requirement of, '…as long as someone speaks my language'. The authors of this paper acknowledge that the process of communication influences each aspect of maternity care and cannot do justice in adding to the 'communication debate' in this paper. However, the message to the reader is that women referred to aspects of communication in a number of ways. A few directly, but more indirectly and often associated with other factors such as preferences for carers, a perceived value of information and the quality of carers interpersonal skills, eg. attentive, 'good' listeners', 'good' at understanding. In addition, when women reflected upon their care, positive and negative experiences were dependent upon the effectiveness of the communication process.

Pregnancy-related locus of control

It is plausible that having insight into women's pregnancy-related locus of control, ie. the extent to which women believe they can influence their own health, could help to explain women's views of and preferences for maternity care. In this study, women completed the Fetal Health Locus of Control scale as described by Labs and Wurtele (1986) and data were compared between ethnic groups. The expectation was that women who scored high on the 'internal' dimension of the scale would score low on one or both of the 'external' scales, or vice versa. And it was anticipated that patterns could be related to women's preferences and views of their care.

Table 9.8: A comparison of the mean FHLC scores for all women, indigenous 'white' and Pakistani women

	All women (n=153)	Indigenous 'white' women (n=77)	Pakistani women (n=76)
'Internal'	43 (10.4) *45*	39 (10.9) *40*	47 (7.8) *50*
'Powerful others'	27 (16.9) *25*	18 (12) *18*	37 (15.3) *42*
'Chance'	41 (14.9) *46*	33 (15.2) *33*	49 (8.6) *54*

(Differences between ethnic groups: Mann-Whitney U test: 'Internal' U=1453, P<.001, 'Chance' U=905, P<.001, 'Powerful others' U=986, P<.001)

These results suggest that although both groups of women assumed responsibility for their un-born baby's health, external factors appeared to have an important influence, particularly for Pakistani women who clearly believed that health carers and the play of chance had an important effect. It was unexpected to find that overall, women scored high on both the 'internal' and 'chance' (external) sub-scales and low on the 'powerful others' sub-scale. This pattern was most noticeable for indigenous 'white' women, whereas Pakistani women scored high on both the external (particularly 'chance') and 'internal' sub-scales. It was highly significant that Pakistani women consistently scored higher than indigenous 'white' women on each of the sub-scales (Mann-Whitney U test: 'internal'— U=1453, P<.001, 'chance' — U=905, P<.001, 'powerful others'—U=986, P<.001). An explanation for this could be that one of the questions referred to the influence of 'God' and, generally, religion plays a more significant role in the lives of Pakistani women than indigenous 'white' women.

For all women the correlation between the 'internal' and both 'powerful others' and 'chance' sub-scales were positive ('internal' and 'powerful others' — rho=.58, P<.001 and 'internal' and 'chance' — rho=.36, P<.001). However, these overall results disguise the different patterns within ethnic groups. For indigenous 'white' women, the relationship between the internal and external sub-scales was conflicting. There was a negative correlation, but not significant, between the 'internal' and 'chance' sub-scales (rho=-.15, P=.19), which is in the expected direction, yet almost no relationship between 'internal' and 'powerful others' sub-scales (rho=.09, P=.4). For Pakistani women the pattern was different. There was a positive relationship between both the 'internal' and 'chance' and, particularly, the 'internal' and 'powerful others' sub-scales ('internal' and 'chance' — rho=.44, P<.001, and 'powerful others' — rho= .71, P<.001).

It was plausible that differences between the ethnic groups could have been caused by the translation and interpretation of the FHLC scale. Therefore, Pakistani women who had their interview translated were compared to those who did not. Within English speaking Pakistani women the same contradictory pattern persisted with women scoring high on both the 'internal' and 'chance' sub-scale and low on the 'powerful others' sub-scale. For non-English speaking women a more even profile was found as non-English speaking Pakistani women consistently scored significantly higher on each of the sub-scales than English speaking Pakistani women (Mann-Whitney U test: 'internal'— U=279, P<.001, 'chance' — U=255, P<.001, 'powerful others'— U=259, P<.001). For Pakistani women who did not speak English the relationship between the 'internal' and the 'powerful others' sub-scale was again positively correlated and significant (rho=.68, P<001); for Pakistani women spoke English the relationship was similar but not as significant (rho=.49, P=.01).

The question still remained whether this finding was a feature of the translation and interpretation process, the effect of two interviewers or effects that could be culturally determined. Data were explored to see whether differences existed between indigenous 'white' women and English speaking Pakistani women. A similar contradictory pattern was found, in that both groups scored high on the 'internal' and 'chance' sub-scale and low on the 'powerful others'. There were no significant differences found within the 'internal' sub-scale but there were between both external sub-scales, Pakistani women scoring higher in both cases (Mann-Whitney U test: 'chance' — U=570.5, P=.001, 'powerful others'— U=6888, P=.017). This analysis confirmed that the pattern was consistent for English speaking women from both ethnic groups.

It was anticipated that patterns of locus of control, identified at group level, would affect women's preferences and views of their care. Although the expected patterns of pregnancy-related locus of control scale were not found in either ethnic group, associations were drawn between group FHLC scores and group analysis of women's preferences and views. In particular, it was observed that Pakistani women, who accepted that all three sub-scales were important, were more flexible in their preferences around the frequency of antenatal visits and for professional types (as long as other conditions were satisfied, such as gender and professional competency). Also, women who believed that they were equally responsible for their un-born baby's health in conjunction with health professionals and the play of chance, viewed the maternity services as complementary rather than essential. This could explain, what appears to be, a relaxed attitude towards carers for some women.

For indigenous 'white' women, associations were found in that FHLC scores suggested that they believed that health professionals were less important to the health of their unborn baby and generally commented more negatively about the care that they received. It cannot be assumed, however, that these findings are strongly related, but it was noted that women who assumed responsibility in conjunction with the play of chance upon the health of their un-born baby were more critical of the service that they received.

In summary, the results from the FHLC scale revealed a number of unexpected findings. In particular, we did not find the expected patterns of women reporting a high 'internal' and low 'external' locus of control or vice versa in either ethnic group. It was found that the relationship between the 'internal' and 'powerful others' sub-scale differed as indigenous 'white' women who had a high 'internal' score reported a low 'powerful others' score, whereas Pakistani women viewed both 'internal' and 'powerful others' as being important. In fact, Pakistani women were found to accept a strong personal responsibility for the health of their un-born baby in conjunction with their professional carers and accepted that there was the influence of 'chance'. Indigenous 'white' women were less strong in their view, overall they accepted their own responsibility but viewed 'chance' as having a greater effect than that of professional carers.

The contradictory results of women assuming personal responsibility and 'chance' as important influences is a concern, as such conflicting beliefs are likely to influence women's views of the quality of their care and possibly the dietary and lifestyle choices that women make whilst they are pregnant.

The usefulness of using the FHLC scale for women in the UK, particularly women from lower social groups, needs further investigation. Also, the validity of translating the FHLC scale into Urdu script and then from Urdu to Punjabi dialect was unclear and it was a concern that the translated interview scores were mainly high. There are a number of plausible explanations for this outcome. It is possible that two interviewers had an unexpected effect or that the translation process was flawed or perhaps non-English speaking Pakistani women generally held strong views, ie. they either strongly agreed or strongly disagreed with a statement. Other literature has questioned the concept of the 'internal' and 'external' locus of control and the appropriateness of using locus of control scales amongst Asian women because of different cultural beliefs, particularly around the influence of religion (Wrightson and Wardle, 1997).

To conclude, this chapter offers a practical and manageable insight into the way in which maternity care can be assessed for women from two ethnic groups in different districts. It also offers 'missing data' from the body of knowledge around women's views of maternity services. It is anticipated that women's views of their maternity care will continue to be explored and underpin quality assessments and strategic planning. Obtaining the views of women is not complex; it requires careful planning and an inherent respect for the participants who agree to take part.

References

Ahmad WUI (1989) Policies, pills and political will: A critique of policies to improve the health status of ethnic minorities. *The Lancet* **1**: 148–50

Balarajan R, Raleigh V (1993) *Ethnicity and Health: A Guide to the NHS*. HMSO, London

Bielawska-Batorowicz E (1993) The effect of previous obstetric history on women's scores on the fetal health locus of control scale (FHLC). *J Reprod Infant Psychol* **11**: 103–6

Bowes AM, Domokos TM (1996) Pakistani women and maternity care: raising muted voices. *Soc Health Illness* **18**: 45–65

Burnard P (1991) A method of analysing interview transcripts in qualitative research. *Nurse Educ Today* **11**: 451–66

Confidential Enquiry into Maternal Deaths (2001) *Why Mothers Die 1997–1999. Report on confidential enquiries into maternal deaths in the United Kingdom.* RCOG Press, London

Department of Health (1993) *Report of the Expert Maternity Group, Part 1 'Changing Childbirth'*. HMSO, London

Donabedian A (1992) Quality assurance in healthcare: consumers' role. *Quality in Healthcare* **1**(4): 247–51

Field PA, Morse JM (1992) *Nursing Research: The application of qualitative approaches*. Chapman Hall, London

Garcia J, Redshaw M, Fitzsimons B, Keene J (1998) *First Class Delivery: A national survey of women's views of maternity care*. National Perinatal Epidemiology Unit, Oxford

Green JM, Coupland VA, Kitzinger JV (1990) Expectations, experiences and psychological outcomes of childbirth: A prospective study of 825 women. *Birth* **17**(1): 15–24

Gready M, Newburn M, Gauge S (1995) *Birth Choices: Women's expectations and experiences*. National Childbirth Trust, London

Hemingway H, Saunders D, Parsons L (1994) *Women's experiences of maternity Services in East London: An Evaluation*. Directorate of Public Health, East London and the City Health Authority, London

Hill AM, Yudkin PL, Bull DJ, Barlow DH, Charnock FM, Gillmer MD (1993) Evaluating a policy of reduced consultant antenatal clinic visits for low risk multiparous women. *Quality in Health Care* **2**: 152–6

Hirst J, Dowswell T, Hewison J, Lilford (1996) Women's views of their first antenatal visit. *Br J Gen Pract* **46**: 319

Hirst J, Hewison J, Kauser Z (1998) *Assessing the Quality of the Maternity Services for Pakistani Women and Indigenous White Women*. Report to the Northern and Yorkshire Region. Centre of Reproduction Growth and Development, University of Leed

Hirst J, Hewison J (2001) Pakistani and indigenous 'white' women's views and the Donabedian-Maxwell grid: a consumer focused template for assessing the quality of maternity care. *Int J Health Care Quality Assurance* **14**(7): 308–16

Hirst J, Hewison J (2002) Hospital postnatal care: obtaining the views of Pakistani and indigenous 'white' women. *Clin Effectiveness Nurs* **6**: 10–18

House of Commons Health Committee (2003a) *Inequalities in Access to Maternity Services*. Eighth report of session 2002–2003. The Stationery Office, London

House of Commons Health Committee (2003b) *Choice in Maternity Services*. Ninth report of session 2002–2003. The Stationery Office, London.

Labs SM, Wurtele SK (1986) Fetal health locus of control scale: development and validation. *J Consult Clin Psychol* **54**(6): 814–19

Macfarlane A, Mugford M (1984) *Birth Counts: statistics of pregnancy and childbirth*. HMSO, London

Martin-Hirsch J, Wright G (1998) The development of a quality model: measuring effective midwifery services. *Int J Health Care Quality Assurance* **11**(2): 50–7

Mays N, Pope C (1996) *Qualitative Research in Healthcare*. British Medical Journal Publishing Group, London

Maxwell RJ (1992) Dimensions of quality revisited: from thought to action. *Quality Health Care* **1**: 171–7

Moser CA, Kalton G (1996) *Survey Methods in Social Investigation*. 2nd edn. Dartmouth Publishing Co, Hants

National Institute for Clinical Excellence (2003) *Antenatal Care: routine care for the healthy pregnant women*. NICE, London.

Ogden J, Shaw A, Zander L (1998) Women's experience of having a hospital birth. *Br J Midwif* **6**(5): 339–45

Proctor S, Wright G (1998) Consumer responses to health care: women and maternity services. *Int J Health Care Quality Assurance* **11**(5): 147–55

Porter M, MacIntyre S (1984) What is, must be best: a research note on conservative or differential responses to antenatal care provision. *Soc Sci Med* **19**: 1197–200

Quine L, Rutter DR, Gowen S (1993) Women's satisfaction with the quality of the birth experience: a prospective study of social and psychological predictors. *J Reprod Infant Psychol* **11**: 107–13

Richens Y (2003) *Exploring the Experiences of Women of Pakistani Origin of UK Maternity Services*. Department of Health, London

Rudat K, Roberts C, Chowdhury R (1993) *Maternity Services: A Comparative Survey of Afro-Caribbean, Asian and White Women*. Market and Opinion Research. International Health Research, London

Shiekh K, Theodore-Ghandi B (1988) *Maternity Service Consumer Survey Report*. Bradford Health Authority, Bradford

Schott J, Henly A (1996) *Culture, Religion and Childbearing in a Multiracial Society*. Butterworth Heinemann, London

Spirito A, Ruggiero L, McGarvey ST, Coustan DR, Graff-Low K (1990) Maternal and fetal health locus of control during pregnancy: A comparison of women with diabetes and non diabetic women. *J Reprod Infant Psychol* **8**: 195–206

Tew M (1990) *Safer Childbirth*. Chapman Hall, London

Tinsley BJ, Trupin SR, Owens L, Boyen LA (1993) The significance of women's pregnancy-related locus of control beliefs for adherence to recommended Prenatal health regimes and pregnancy outcomes. *J Reprod Infant Psychol* **11**: 97–102

Townsend P, Davidson N (1982) *Inequalities in Health: The Black Report*. Pelican, London

Whitehead M (1987) *The Health Divide: Inequalities in Health in the 1980s*. Health Education Council, London

Williams B (1994) Patient satisfaction: a valid concept? *Soc Sci Med* **38**(4): 509–16

Woollett A, Dosanhj N, Nicolson P, Marshall H, Djhanbakhch O, Hadlow J (1995) The ideas and experiences of pregnancy and childbirth of Asian and non-Asian women in east London. *Br J Med Psychol* **68**: 65–84

Wrightson KJ, Wardle J (1997) Culture variation in health locus of control. *Ethnicity Health* **2**(12): 13–20

10

How stereotyping can lead to ineffective care and treatment: Pakistani women's experiences of UK maternity services: a case study

Yana Richens

The aim of this chapter is to challenge any assumptions and stereotypical beliefs that midwives may hold of certain client groups. Stereotyping has been defined as making inaccurate judgements or assumptions about an individual in a whole group based on the supposed characteristic of that group (Allport, 1954). The major problem with stereotyping is that it reduces people to one aspect of their identity. In the case of Asian women this may be that they are quiet, reserved and often do not speak English. The difficulty with this is that it presents a homogenous view of Asian women, which in reality is not the case.

Stereotyping of certain groups of people can and does lead to major failures in the delivery of care to particular client groups (Bennett Inquiry, 2004). Some have suggested it has led to institutionalised racism, which has been described as a *'festering abscess of the National Health Service'* [NHS] (Carvel, 2004). Institutionalised racism has been defined as:

> *The collective failure of an organisation to provide an appropriate*
> *and professional service to people because of their colour, culture,*
> *or ethnic origin. It can be seen or detected in processes, attitudes*
> *and behaviour which amount to discrimination through unwitting*
> *prejudice, ignorance, thoughtlessness and racist stereotyping which*
> *disadvantage ethnic minority people.*

(MacPherson, 1999)

Studies have highlighted how institutionalised racism can negatively effect communication between women and healthcare professionals in maternity services and how this can lead to substandard care (Bowler, 1993; Bowes and Domokos, 1996; Garcia *et al*, 1998; Rocheron, 1988; McLeish, 2002).

While it may be argued that institutionalised racism is rarely intentional, its effects are devastating. Such devastating effects were recently highlighted by the independent inquiry into the death of David (Rocky) Bennett, a young black man who had been diagnosed with schizophrenia. Rocky Bennett died in 1998 after being restrained by five nurses whilst he was a patient in a psychiatric hospital. The inquiry confirmed publicly that institutionalised racism is present in the NHS and that the NHS fails to provide ethnic minority communities with the services that they require and deserve (Bennett Inquiry, 2004). The authors went further and commented that:

> *Once it is fully recognised by everyone in the NHS that patients'*
> *needs include cultural, social and spiritual needs, real progress can*
> *be made at eradicating institutionalised racism.*

(Bennett Inquiry, 2004: 47)

Rocky Bennett had been stereotyped as a 'black and dangerous' black man, which is not an uncommon stereotype of black male psychiatric patients, a stereotype that is well documented. Dadabhoy (2001) recalls a time when he was called to admit a young black male patient who had been detained under the mental health act for stealing an ice cream, the man was brought to the ward handcuffed and escorted by six policemen, even though the police admitted that he had offered no resistance and had not been violent in anyway. The man was pinned face down on the floor of the examination room and taunted about his sexuality by the officers (2001: 66).

Negative stereotyping in healthcare does not just happen in relation to ethnic minority groups, commentators have reported how it manifests itself in the less favourable treatment of disabled people (Bailey, 1994), lesbians (Platzer, 1993), and individuals with learning difficulties (Brown *et al,* 1994). An ethnographic study undertaken by Bowler (1993) investigated the midwifery care of women from a South Asian descent. Women in the study were labelled and stereotyped as 'all the same' and 'not like us' by midwives and, as a consequence, the care provided to these women was based on the stereotypical beliefs held by the midwives. The study revealed that midwives held a number of negative stereotypes of Asian women, these were that Asian women had difficulty in communicating, they lacked compliance with care given, they abused the service, they lacked any maternal instinct, and they had a tendency to make a fuss about nothing. Bowler (1993) reported how the stereotypical view of Asian women held by midwives affected the midwife-client interaction. For example, if an Asian woman in labour makes a noise it is not because she is in pain, but because Asian women in general have low pain thresholds. In addition, Bowler (1993) also suggests that the stereotypical views held by midwives also extended to Caucasian mothers. Women from a large council estate were described as 'thick'. However, Bowler also pointed out that ethnicity was more important than class when framing stereotypes

In Bowler's study women of South Asian descent were regarded as a homogenous group by the midwives caring for them, despite the fact that the women were heterogeneous in terms of culture and religion. These stereotypes were based on the physical appearance of the women. This is not an uncommon practice and was recently reported by Richens (2003), who commented on how a Pakistani woman reported that she is often asked by the receptionist at the local doctors to act as an interpreter for any women who looked Asian and could not speak English (Richens, 2003: 29).

The formidable challenge facing midwives is around their ability to provide care to a diverse and multicultural population. Midwives are being asked to provide a high quality service that is acceptable to all women. Research has shown that women from whatever socio-economic background or culture want the same thing: good communication, useful information, respect and choice (Richens, 2003; McLeish, 2002; Garcia *et al*, 1998). However, research has also shown that many women from different cultures and lower socio-economic groups do not appear to receive the same amount of communication, information or choice as Caucasian women (Lowe *et al*, 2004; Bowler, 1993). Following the recent death of David Bennett, the Blofeld Inquiry (2004) stated that:

Black and ethnic minority citizens should not have to claim their rights, they should be given them as a matter of course. They are not demanding more than they are entitled to, nor are they claiming preferential treatment. They are simply asking for justice, which has been denied them for too long.

As previously discussed negative stereotypes are one reason why there are variations in care provided to women from different ethnic minority groups and women from lower socio-economic groups. However, variations in care may also be compounded by a lack of time and resources available to midwives. Furthermore, midwives, and the organisations they work for, need to acknowledge that communication with a non-English speaking woman will take longer because of the need for a translation and interpretation of the clinical episode.

Research has shown there is a growing evidence base that women from ethnic minority groups are seldom satisfied with the care they receive (Homans, 1980; Currer, 1986; Dobson, 1986; Cochrane, 1996; Parsons and Day, 1992; Katbamna, 2000; Hirst and Hewison, 2001). Women's experiences may be subject to a range of factors that impact on the quality of care, access and information they receive. However, there is a gap in the literature in that we do not know enough about women's actual experiences of maternity care. The literature review undertaken by Richens (2003) as part of her exploration into Pakistani women's experiences of UK maternity services, identified priorities and factors that may contribute to how Pakistani women experience maternity services, and also highlighted a need for more research exploring women's experience of maternity services.

Tackling Health Inequalities (DoH, 2001) highlights the role of midwives in reducing health inequalities. Before this can realistically happen, however, midwives need to know and they need to understand the problems that are experienced by ethnic minority women when they make use of UK maternity services. A recent report by McKenzie (2003: 66) suggested that:

> *A deeper understanding of possible links between racism and health*
> *is a prerequisite for initiatives to decrease impact at a community*
> *and individual level.*

Hundt (2002) has argued that:

> *Without communication skills to take a good history and without*
> *trust between health professionals and users, a clinician is just a*
> *technician. The ability to integrate different kinds of knowledge,*
> *to problem solve, to place the individual experiences of the local*
> *patient within the social context and global clinical developments are*
> *essential.*

✱ However, we must acknowledge the fact that communication is a two-way process. If a client is unable to understand what is being said, an exchange of information cannot take place — leading to the potential for confused communication and ineffective care and advice. These kind of things can be seen clearly in an interaction reported by Bowler (1993) when a woman was asked about her intended family planning practice after the birth of her fourth baby.

Midwife:	*Do you want more children?*
Woman:	*[confusion]*
Midwife:	*You know, any more babies?*
Woman:	*Four children*
Midwife:	*More babies? Do you want five babies?*
Woman:	*Not five babies, four babies*
Midwife:	*Well go and see Dr Smith in five weeks with your husband and discuss not having any more babies.*

(Bowler, 1993: 165)

In addition to the confusion resulting from poor communication, midwives may also misinterpret positive non-verbal cues, for example, where a women is smiling this may be (wrongly) interpreted that she has understood what has been said to her.

Research exploring the experiences of ethnic minority women provides some insight into the problems associated with communication, information and education and provides some ideas about what effective communication means to women and what happens when communication is not so effective (Clarke and Clayton, 1983; Currer, 1986; Thomas *et al*, 1991; Bowler, 1993; Garcia *et al*, 1998; Gissler *et al*, 1998; Bradby, 2001; Hirst and Hewison, 2001; Petrou *et al*, 2001; McLeish, 2002). Some commentators argue that language, culture and the ethnic origin of women and their carers does have an effect on communication (Currer, 1986; Bowler, 1993; Narang and Murphy, 1994; McLeish, 2002; Richens, 2003).

In an exploration of Pakistani women's experiences of UK maternity services, Richens (2003) divided communication into four sub-themes: explanation, support, behaviour, and skills of the midwife. Here they will all be discussed collectively. The study revealed that it was very important to women that they received good clear explanations of what was going to happen to them. It also was clear how women felt when they did not receive a clear explanation — they reported feeling scared and lonely. While many of the women recognised that communication was a two-way process and that they had a part to play, they nevertheless reported that they seldom asked any questions. However, this was often due to the fact that they could not speak English and did not have an interpreter present. On those occasions when women did ask questions or asked for clarification, they felt that they did not always receive a satisfactory response. For example, one women reported:

> *I was asking her* [the midwife] *questions, but she wouldn't really answer them. I can't remember what I asked her, but it was like yes, no,* [and she] *just walked off.*

> (Richens, 2003: 26)

Women reported further deficiencies in communication when they were left alone during labour or during other unfamiliar situations:

> *After I had the baby I was left in the bathroom on my own for a long time. My husband was not there and I was bleeding a lot, no one came, I was crying and frightened.*

> (Richens, 2003: 26)

Women described how they felt some of the midwives were not 'nice', and the following quotes highlight what women meant by this:

> *... the first time, there was two of them I think with me in the room when I was having the baby. They were just so horrible, you know? They didn't talk to me properly, I was crying and in a lot of pain. They were cruel in the way they were talking to me, they were really horrible...*

> (Richens, 2003: 27)

When asked to clarify further what she meant by horrible, the woman explained:

> *I was panicking and in a lot of pain, I didn't understand what was happening. It's the first baby and you don't know, you just think, what is happening? You shout some, and scream some, and I was shouting and they didn't understand that I was in pain. They were just, like... you know, when you tell someone off?*

> (Richens, 2003: 27)

None of these findings are new, and as discussed above all, women, regardless of colour, background, age or race have similar feelings during labour, and they all want effective communication, information, access and choice.

In an exploration of the attitudes and experiences of Asian women receiving postnatal care (Wollett and Dosanjh-Matwala, 1990) the authors highlight how one woman reported how she was unable to change her baby's nappy:

> *I couldn't do it, I couldn't move. The behaviour of the nurses was*
> *really bad, that's why I ran home. I left the hospital before time. If you*
> *needed anything, they'd talk to you very rudely and not listen to you.*

(p. 182)

In a postal survey of 1188 women (Singh and Newburn, 2000) found that one in five women worried about being left alone during labour. Historically women have always valued a trusting relationship with other women, and this reaches a peak during childbirth (Kitzinger, 2000). Furthermore, psycho-social support given to women during labour has been shown to reduce obstetric interventions and provide women with a more positive childbirth experience (Ryding *et al*, 1998; Enkin *et al*, 1995).

What is new about Richens' (2003) findings, however, is that women who had learned to speak and communicate in English following their first pregnancy, reported that in their second pregnancy they were treated differently — they were treated better. The reasons they gave for this difference in treatment was because they would be able to report the actions of midwives:

> *Before they thought I can't speak English, I can't tell anyone.*

(Richens, 2003: 26)

However, it could be proposed that because the women were now able to understand English there was less opportunity for confusion.

Women also appeared to associate kindness with physical support, so anything that involved touch and hands-on care, practical demonstrations, and being spoken to were viewed positively by the women:

> *The second time I was so pleased. The midwives that I had were*
> *really, really nice. They stayed with me, they were holding my arms,*
> *they were calming, they were talking to me so I didn't think about the*
> *pain, asking, did I have kids, where's your husband?*

(Richens, 2003: 26)

The way in which women responded positively to physical support suggests it is the interpersonal skills of the midwife, including the use of verbal and non-verbal cues that enhances the experience for non-English speaking women. This means that even if an interpreter is not present for any period of time, the women's experience does not have to be a negative one. Further evidence supports this and suggests that women value a midwife who is kind and who respects them, regardless of colour, class or ethnic origin (Langer *et al*, 1993). In an Australian study exploring the views of Vietnamese, Turkish, and Filipino women giving birth in Australia (Small *et al*, 1999) the authors report that women were not concerned that caregivers knew little about their cultural practices, they were more concerned that the care they experienced was unkind, rushed and unsupportive. Similar findings were reported by Garcia *et al* (1998), who commented that:

> *Unfortunately, women's comments often refer to the absence of kindness — of being ignored, told off or criticised. Good care is also care that feels safe and competent, and that includes good communication.*

(Garcia *et al*, 1998: 63)

What must be borne in mind when we are talking about good communication with non-English speaking women is that this can be very different to an English speaking woman born in the UK. For example, what may seem, from the midwife's point of view, to be a very clear and specific request, to a non-English speaking woman, may not be interpreted as such. This is illustrated in the next quote which is an exchange between an interpreter and a non-English speaking Pakistani woman in her late twenties. The situation that is described took place when the woman was thirty-six weeks pregnant with her fifth baby, she had been experiencing reduced fetal movements and had made an appointment to see her midwife at her GP's surgery:

Woman: *I told her* [midwife]. *Then she said to me go to the hospital, but I went two weeks later.*

Interpreter: *So you went two weeks later, did the midwife not tell you to go straight away?*

Woman: *Yes, if you can go.*

Interpreter: *Didn't the midwife tell you that this was a serious matter, that you had to go now?*

Woman: *I felt scared; I was scared that I would need a caesarean section.*

Interpreter: *Was there anyone to explain all this to you?*

Woman: *No.*

Interpreter: *When you went to the hospital after two weeks what did they do?*

Woman: *They attached me to a machine, and it didn't seem right, and they gave me some medicine.*

Interpreter: *After the baby was born, did they explain to you what the problem was?*

Woman: *No nothing, and when the baby was born the cord was wrapped round his neck.*

When asked why the woman delayed going to the hospital, the woman again said she had been scared. However, it also became clear that she did not realise the implications and the possible consequences of what had been said to her:

> Interpreter: *When the midwife told you, you got scared, you didn't go, what could have been done to make you less scared?*
>
> Woman: *I think that if I did go, who would look after my other children?*

When asked by the interpreter what she would do if it happened again, the woman went on to say:

> Woman: *I would go to the hospital first, I do not want any more children, I'm scared after having this baby, I'm really terrified.*
>
> Interpreter: *What do you think can be done to stop this happening to anyone else?*
>
> Woman: *I don't know what to tell you. They should go to the hospital and get it checked.*
>
> Interpreter: *No, no, that's fine... Do you feel that it was explained properly?*
>
> Woman: *I thought that there was only two weeks left until the baby was to be born.*

The baby born to this woman was barely alive and now has severe physical and mental development problems. To prevent a similar situation occurring there are two major things to consider. First, the role of the midwife in the antenatal situation and what her actions could and should have been, and second, the actions of the woman. There needs to be some way of checking the process of understanding. If someone does not speak the same language then ensuring that a correct interpretation of what has been said, which takes into account conceptual equivalence, cultural interpretation and understanding, is an essential part of the communication process. Midwives must be made aware of these cases and the impact that ineffective communication can have on the lives of these women and their families. It would appear, however, that many midwives are not aware of the significant impact that effective communication can have on a woman and her family's life. One solution to these difficulties in communication may be to make greater use of link workers or health advocates to translate information for the woman and to ensure that the woman fully understands.

It is also equally important that members of the family are not used as translators since this has been reported as being distressing for both the woman and the person being asked to translate. Using family members or other Asian speakers who may be neighbours clearly contravenes confidentiality. For example, if a midwife suspects a woman is a victim of domestic violence and she relies on the woman's husband or her mother-in-law to act as an interpreter it is very unlikely that the women will be able to confide in the midwife. Research has shown that mothers do not like keeping their children off school to act as interpreters (Narang and Murphy, 1994). The following quote was a memory recalled by one woman who had been kept home from school as a child to interpret for her mother. This episode still appeared to cause her some concern, as she faltered when talking about this:

> *It would have been better if mother had had a proper interpreter as I didn't really understand what they* (midwives) *were telling me, and mum seemed upset.*

(Richens, 2003: 29)

Women also reported how their husbands were commonly cited as being asked to interpret for them during labour. While this was acceptable for some of the women, such acceptance needs to be placed within a cultural framework. For other women having their husbands act as an interpreter caused problems because they felt their husbands were selective in what they interpreted. For example:

> *... he never explains properly he just says, 'ah I know they said this and that,' ... he just kept saying, 'you are fine, you are fine'. Because he goes to work and then he comes back home to pick me up and we go to the surgery, then he goes back to work and it is hard for him as well.*

(Richens, 2003: 29)

In addition, several of the women reported that it was inappropriate when they were asked by healthcare staff to act as interpreters for other women even when they did not speak the same language. Such requests were made in hospitals and in GP surgeries. For example:

> *She* [woman] *was in a lot of pain and the nurses were asking her where your pain is, and she was trying to tell them, but she was angry at the same time. I said it to her although she was a Bengali speaker, I said 'she is asking where is your pain?', and she said, 'here by the side'.... it is really frustrating I mean, she was in agony.*

(Richens, 2003: 29)

Another woman reported:

> *... many times I have been down the surgery and at reception someone is giving their name and everything, then the receptionist asks me, 'cos I look like an Asian, they say to me 'you explain to her what I am saying'.*

(Richens, 2003: 29)

Some of the women who had been asked to translate were unhappy about these requests: they felt that they were being involved in something that was private and confidential. They also felt that there might be some ramifications for them on a personal level, that they might be labelled as gossips. Furthermore, they believed that some women had been treated unjustly, even missing appointments because of the lack of interpreters. For example, one woman reported:

> ... *I was in the surgery and there was a family there from Libya and the lady was pregnant, she didn't understand English and she was waiting for an interpreter to come, but the interpreter was a bit late so the woman lost her appointment at the surgery.*

(Richens, 2003: 30)

One way of supporting midwives in delivering good competent care to women whose first language is not English is the provision of good information. Pakistani women often require good information even before they conceive, and this should continue throughout the antenatal, birth and postnatal periods. Richens (2003) found that women reported a need for information that was available in the appropriate language and format. In addition to this, and the need for written information, the women also suggested the provision of videos or audio tapes. These types of resources need to be made available to midwives, and are crucial if maternity care is to be based upon the best available evidence, to enable women to become partners in their care. As one woman explained:

> *Honestly it was really hard; I never used to understand what they were saying. I used to cry. They would write it down on paper for me to show to my husband and then he used to explain it to me hours later.*

(Richens, 2003: 30)

Other women when referring to the hand-held green antenatal records (a complete record of their antenatal care) said:

> *'I may as well have had a blank piece of paper'; 'I never understood what they were on about, I used to go home and cry my head off, I did not know what they were saying'; 'I just looked at the pictures and thought that looks awful.'*

(Richens, 2003: 30)

The inability to understand the information they were given was not restricted to the antenatal period, it also occurred during the postnatal period. During one of the focus groups women discussed the importance of contraception and the associated information they had been given, with some women reporting how they felt this was culturally inappropriate:

*You were given this leaflet with, this penis sticking out. What does
that mean to an Asian woman?*

(Richens, 2003: 30)

A recent study by Lowe *et al* (2004) highlighted the lack of provision of written
information in the appropriate language, and drew attention to the way in which
women appeared to accept poor treatment as the norm. For example, Lowe *et al*
(2004) report how South Asian women did not realise that it is not acceptable
for doctors to shout at patients. Research has shown that women also want
more, and better, information on maternity services and contraception (Garcia
et al, 1998; Singh and Newburn, 2000). A study exploring the provision of
maternity information (Schonveld and Kingswell, 1996) actively sought out
the views of black and ethnic minority women, women with disabilities and
young single women. The findings show that women identified two main
areas of concern: the lack of information available in the appropriate language;
and difficulties understanding maternity terminology (even for those women
who spoke English). This again reinforces the idea that women themselves,
regardless of their background, want relevant, understandable and accessible
information.

Choice for non-English speaking women is meaningless unless the
language barrier is broken down. However, choice continues to be the mantra
for modern maternity services, and public declarations of the need for choice
are not uncommon, as evidenced by a quote from Yvette Cooper, Minister for
Health, given at a National Childbirth conference:

*Women and their partners need proper choices in maternity care
and childbirth. Every woman has their own views about the kind of
support they want during childbirth. Some want a home birth, others
want epidurals and rapid pain relief.*

(Cooper, 2001)

The reality is that ethnic minority women often do not get a choice, and this is
extended to other services. Lowe *et al* (2004), in a study exploring the barriers
to services for South Asian women seeking contraception, found that women
were provided with insufficient information by health professionals, they
were subjected to paternalistic attitudes by doctors, and they had no sense of
entitlement which could lead to them becoming empowered. These women
were refused sterilisations and terminations and they were also discouraged and
berated for using emergency contraception (Lowe *et al*, 2004).

However, in some areas the concept of choice is an alien concept, and
what is viewed as a positive choice in the UK, may not be construed as such in
another country. For example, a home birth is something that many women in
the UK aspire to, while in other countries it is seen as an indicator of a woman's
poverty. As such, having the opportunity for a hospital birth is an excellent
choice for a lot of non-English speaking women. Richens (2003) reported how

two women who had given birth at home in Pakistan, said that they would not consider it in the UK. They recalled their experience of giving birth in Pakistan as very positive, they had been attended by the local midwife and they had been supported by female relatives. However, husbands were excluded from being present, and for one woman this was a negative experience and she had preferred having a hospital birth in the UK because her husband could stay with her. However, having a hospital birth was not without its problems. Some women felt that the hospital bureaucracy both prevented and affected their own social support systems (Richens, 2003). They cited restrictive visiting times, not being able to have more than one person present in the labour room, midwives acting as gatekeepers and not informing relatives who telephoned for information. These were seen as negative factors in giving birth in hospital, but the women still expressed reservations about giving birth at home.

Antenatal education provoked both positive and negative discussion, and general comments included inappropriate times and locations of classes, which acted as a barrier to attendance. The women felt that if the time of classes were changed then it would be possible for their husbands to attend also. Others reported that they had attended classes in their second pregnancy and they found this helpful, although some reported not being able to attend local classes:

> When I had the other children there were no classes whatsoever and I think I really needed the support then, you know every pregnancy is different and you are scared.

(Richens, 2003: 31)

Classes served a dual purpose in that they provided the women with an opportunity to see the midwife and ask questions. However, the women did not identify a need for classes to be organised in different languages.

Generally the women reported a positive experience in terms of their postnatal care compared to antenatal care and birth experiences. However, they did report that their religious choices were not always considered following the birth of their baby, since they were often not given any opportunity to perform religious ceremonies. After birth it is the custom for Muslim families to perform the Azaan (call to prayer) on the new-born. These ideally should be the first words to reach the child's ears. For this religious custom to take place the baby needs to be clean. However, for many of the women this was difficult:

> I had a caesarean, and I asked if they could bathe my child 'cos we're gonna have the Azaan, but she [midwife] said to me I will do it later. I said the baby has to be clean and she said to me can't you do it later and I said no 'cos I've invited the molvi to come down today, in the end I just had to persist. Look I want the baby to have a bath and I want it now.

(Richens, 2004: 32)

Several of the women reported how they had been given choice with menu options, although some of them felt that it was occasionally assumed that they would always opt for an Asian meal rather than an English meal. All the women reported that they would have preferred to have stayed in hospital for a longer period of time, even though all of their visitors were not allowed. They felt that they needed more time to rest. The women were generally satisfied with community care in the postnatal period and gave more positive comments about community midwives:

> *She (midwife) is great, she understands that we shave the babies head, and doesn't even mention it.*
>
> (Richens, 2003: 33)

The challenge for maternity services

What has been described above highlights the key challenges that need to be addressed in the delivery of effective maternity services for all women in the twenty-first century. In an amendment to the 1976 Race Relations Act, the Government strengthened the duty placed on all public institutions to prevent discriminating against people on the basis of race (Home Office, 2001). To fulfil the requirements of the amendment, there is a need to provide translation and interpretation services for patients whose first language is not English. The Government has pledged that free translation and interpretation services will be available from all NHS premises by 2003 through NHS Direct (DoH, 2000). Ensuring that translation and interpretation services are available in areas with a population whose first language is not English will go some way in ensuring that these diverse populations are provided with equal opportunities to be involved in decisions about their care and treatment, and in the way services are planned, delivered and evaluated. However, there still appears to be a reluctance to involve interpreters in maternity services, and where interpreters are used there are reports that they are not treated as part of the clinical team. The perceived low status of interpreters has been recognised and suggestions made. For example:

> *I would like to see link-workers enjoy a higher status in the workplace, with a national system of accreditation in place.*
>
> (Payne, 1994: 59)

Midwives need to establish a good working relationship with interpreters, one that is based on mutual trust and respect. An incident report should be completed whenever it is not possible to locate or get in touch with an interpreter. Family, friends, neighbours or strangers should not be asked to act as interpreters, and midwives should strive to ensure that they see a woman at least once in the presence of an interpreter. Other suggestions for the effective use of translation and interpretation services are given in *Box10.1*.

Box 10.1: Key points in the effective use of translation and interpretation services

⌘ When booking an interpreter give as much warning as possible.
⌘ Give precise details about where, when and how long the interpreter is needed.
⌘ Give the name and address of the patient/client.
⌘ Specify the language spoken by the patient/client, not just the nationality (if in doubt, the interpreter should be asked to contact the patient/client).
⌘ Briefly explain the purpose of the consultation.
⌘ Be punctual.
⌘ Book the same interpreter for subsequent visits.
⌘ Address the patient in the second person.
⌘ Talk directly to the patient.
⌘ Keep control of the consultation.
⌘ Pause frequently.
⌘ Appear attentive when patient/client responds.
⌘ Respond to non-verbal clues.
⌘ Check out the patient's/client's understanding of what has been said.
⌘ Allow enough time for the patient/client to ask questions.
⌘ Make use of any available written information.

Adapted from: Phelan and Parkman (1995)

In terms of communication midwives must constantly ensure that the instructions she is giving to the client are understood. Time should be taken to allow the woman to ask clarifying questions, if necessary through ensuring that a translator is present. Given the findings reported above, midwives should also remain cautious about relying on family, neighbours or even strangers being asked to interpret. While language may not be everything, it is also important that midwives use appropriate non-verbal communication to reassure constantly and support women.

One way of dealing with cultural differences is to ensure that healthcare professionals are trained to be aware of the specific social, cultural and physical needs of ethnic minority women, something which has previously been overlooked in healthcare education (Chevannes, 2002). This requires a change of focus in terms of greater cultural understanding, and the provision of relevant information and education for ethnic minority women and their families, where they need it, when they need it, and in a form they can understand. When we have achieved that we may start to see a reduction in the perinatal mortality rate in this group of women.

Our failure actively to involve Pakistani women in the planning of care and services, as well as our failure to ask them about their experiences, has been identified as arising from a lack of funding, or a lack of patient satisfaction questionnaires being made available in a variety of different languages. However, it may be equally true that some people remain firmly entrenched in a stereotypical belief that even if these patient satisfaction measures were available, Pakistani women would still not be able to understand them because they are illiterate. However patient/public involvement and participation is a major focus of Government attempts to modernise the NHS over the last decade (DoH, 1997; 1998; 1999; 2001), and is seen as crucial in improving the quality of care for everyone. The *NHS Plan* for England (DoH, 2000) devotes an entire chapter to this. In addition, placing the patients' experiences at the heart of health care is one of the five key elements of clinical governance (RCN, 2003). Strategies to involve non-English speaking women must be tailored to meet their needs and be based on a commitment to equality and participation in the delivery of healthcare services (RCN, 2003). Furthermore, this involvement of women and families in service design and delivery is central to implementing the *National Service Framework for children, young people and maternity services* (DoH, 2004), as maternal health is seen as a continuum of health care

Coulter (2002) has argued that we must start to see things through the patient's eyes and that patient and public involvement needs to be a central element of professional training and continuing development, and is a key challenge for educators and healthcare organisations. The challenge of delivering effective, equitable maternity services is the ultimate challenge for those of us who have a responsibility to deliver care and treatment to a diverse, multicultural population with a wide range of needs.

Learning to see things through a patient's eye should be a central part of professional training and continuing development.

(Coulter 2002: 108)

References

Allport GW (1954) *The Nature of Prejudice*. Addison Wesley, Workingham

Bailey AM (1994) A handicap of negative attitudes and lack of choice: caring for inpatients with disabilities. *Prof Nurs* September: 786–8

Bennett Inquiry (2004) Available online at: http:/wwwimage.guardian.co.uk/sys-files/Society/documents/2004/02/12/Bennett.pdf

Blofeld J (2004) *Guardian* 12 February 2004. Available online at: http://wwwsociety/guardian.co.uk/mentalhealth/story/0,8150,1146748,00html

Bowler I (1993) They're not the same as us: midwives stereotypes of South Asian women. *Sociol Health Illness* **81**(1): 46–65

Bowes AM, Meehan Domokos T (1998) Health visitors' work in a multi-ethnic society: a qualitative study of social exclusion. *J Soc Policy* **27**(4) 489–506

Bradby H (2001) Communication, interpretation and translation. In: Culley L, Dyson S, eds. *Ethnicity and Nursing Practice*. Palgrave, Basingstoke

Brown H, Turke V, Stein J (1994) Sexual abuse of adults with learning difficulties. *Social Care Research Findings* **46**. Joseph Rowntree Foundation, York

Carvel (2004) Abscess of NHS racism exposed. *Guardian*: 6 February. Available online at: http://wwwsociety.guardian.co.uk/mentalhealth/story/0,8150,1142309,00.html (accessed 20 February 2004)

Chevannes M (2002) Issue in education: health professionals to meet the diverse needs of patients and other service users from ethnic minority groups. *J Adv Nurs* **39**(3) 290–8

Clarke M, Clayton D (1983) Quality of obstetric care provided for Asian immigrants in Leicester. *Br Med J* **297**: 384–7

Cochrane R (1996) Women's experience of antenatal care in Tower Hamlets. In: McKie L, ed. *Researching Women Health: methods and processes*. Quay Books, MA Healthcare Limited, Wiltshire:151–75

Cooper Y (2001) Available online at: http://www.dh.gov.uk/Publications AndStatistics/PressReleases/PressReleasesNotices/fs/en?CONTENT_ ID=4010584&chk=%2BzQHq2 (accessed 24 February 2004)

Coulter A (2002) *The Autonomous Patient: Ending Paternalism in Medical Care*. The Nuffield Trust

Currer C (1986) *Health concepts and illness behaviour: the case of some Pathan Mothers in Britain*. PhD Thesis, University of Warwick.

Dadabhoy S (2001) The next generation, the problematic children, a personal story. In: Coker N, ed. *Racism in Medicine: An agenda for change*. King's Fund, London

Department of Health (1993) *Changing Childbirth: Report of the Expert Maternity Group* (Cumberledge Report). HMSO, London

Department of Health (1997) The New NHS — modern, dependable. DoH, London

Department of Health (1998) *A first class service: Quality in the new NHS*. Stationery Office, London

Department of Health (1999) *Saving Lives: Our healthier nation.* Stationery Office, London

Department of Heath (2000) *The NHS Plan: A plan for investment, a plan for reform.* Stationery Office, London

Department of Health (2001) *Tackling Health Inequalities: Consultation on a plan for delivery.* Stationery Office, London

Department of Health (2002a) *NHS trust-based patient surveys: inpatients — acute hospitals.* Stationery Office, London

Department of Health (2002b) *Partnership working.* Available online at: http//:www.doh.gov.uk/prcare/pdfs/nsf_partnershipworking.

Department of Health (2004) *National service framework for children, young people and maternity services.* The Stationary Office, London

Dobson S (1986) Ethnic identity: a basis for care. *Midwife Health Visitor and Comm Nurs* **24**(5): 172

Enkin M, Keirse MJNC, Renfrew M, Neilson JA (1995) *Guide to Effective Care in Pregnancy and Childbirth.* Oxford University Press, Oxford

Garcia J, Redshaw M, Fitzsimons B, Keene J (1998) *First class delivery: a national survey of women's views of maternity care.* Audit Commission. Belmont Press

Gissler M, Woolett M, Geraedts M, Hemminki E, Buekeris P (1998) Insufficient prenatal care in Finland and Baden. Wurttemberg. *Eur J Pub Health* **8**: 227–31

Hennings J, Williams J, Naher, Haque B (1996) Exploring the health needs of Bangladeshi women: a case study in using qualitative research methods. *Health Educ J* **55**: 11–23

Hirst J, Hewison J (2001) Pakistani and indigenous white women's views and the Donabedian Maxwell grid; a consumer-focused template for assessing the quality of maternity care. *Int J Healthc Quality Ass* **14**(7): 308–16

Home Office (2001) Race Relations (Amendment) Act 2000: chapter 34. Available online at: http://www.hmso.gov.uk/acts/acts2000/20000034.htm.

Homans HY (1980) *Pregnant in Britain: a Sociological Approach to Asian and British Women's Experience.* PhD Thesis, University of Warwick.

Hunt SC (2003) *Poverty, Pregnancy and the Health Care Professional.* Elselvier, London

Hundt G (2002) Inaugural lecture: 'Local Voices on Global Health Issues'. 10 September 2002. Warwick University, Warwick

Katbamna S (2000) *Race and Childbirth.* Open University Press, Buckingham

Kitzinger S (2000) *Rediscovering Birth.* Little Brown and Company, St Helens

Langer A, Victora C, Victora M *et al* (1993) The Latin American trial of psychosocial support during pregnancy: a social intervention evaluated though an experimental design. *Soc Sci Med* **36**(4): 495–507

Lowe P, Griffiths F, Sidhu R (2004) A consideration of institutional barriers preventing south Asian women accessing contraceptive service. Presentation of findings at University Hospitals Coventry and Warwickshire Trust, 28 January 2004

Lavender T, Chapple J (2003) *Models of maternity care: Summary of findings*. Available online at: http://www.doh.gov.uk/maternitywg/report-jan03.htm

Macpherson W (Chair) (1999) *The Lawrence Inquiry, vols 1 and 2*. HMSO, London

McKenzie K (2003) Racism and health. *Br Med J* **326**: 65–6

McLeish J (2002) *Mothers in exile — Maternity experiences of asylum seekers in England*. The Maternity Alliance, London

Narang I, Murphy S (1994) Assessment of the antenatal care for Asian women. *Br J Midwifery* **2**(4): 169–73

Parsons L, Day S (1992) Improving obstetric outcomes in ethnic minorities: an evaluation of health advocacy in Hackney. *J Public Health Med* **14**(2): 183–91

Payne S (1994) Mother tongues. *Nursing Times* **90**(26): 59

Petrou S, Kupek K, Vause S, Maresh M (2001) Clinical, provider and socio-demographic determinants of the number of antenatal visits in England and Wales. *Soc Sci Med* **52**: 1123–34

Phelan M, Parkman S (1995) How to do it: Work with an interpreter. *Br Med J* **311**: 555–7

Platzer H (1993) 'Nursing care of gay and lesbian patients'. *Nurs Standard* **7**(17): 34–7

Richens Y (2003) *Exploring the experiences of women of Pakistani origin of UK maternity services*. Available online at: www.yanarichens.com

Rocheron Y, Dickinson R, Kahn S (1988) *Evaluation of the Asian mother and baby campaign*. King's Fund, London

Rowe R, Garcia J, Macfarlane A, Davidson L (1999) Communication issue in stillbirth and infant death: a review of communication within the CESDI Framework. National Perinatal Epidemiology Unit

Royal College of Nursing (2003) *Clinical governance: A resource guide*. RCN, London

Ryding, EL, Wijma B, Wimja K (1998) Fear of childbirth during pregnancy may increase the risk of emergency caesarean. *Acta Obstet Gynecol Scand* **77**(5): 542–7

Schonveld A, Kingswell S (1996) *Improving Maternity Information — A Consultation Process*. Project report, Coventry Health Promotion Services, Coventry

Singh, D Newburn M (2000) *Access to Maternity Information and Support — The experiences and needs of women before and after giving birth*. NCT, London

Small R, Liamputtong RP, Yelland J, Lumley J (1999) Mother in a new country. The role of culture and communication in Vietnamese, Turkish and Filipino women's experiences of giving birth in Australia. *Women and Health* **28**(3), Hawthorne Press

Thomas P, Golding J, Peters TJ (1991) Delayed antenatal care: does it affect pregnancy outcome? *Soc Sci Med* **32**: 714–23

White P, Philips K, Minns A (1999) *Women from ethnic minority communities: Their knowledge of and needs for health advocacy services in east London*. Staffordshire Press, Stoke-on-Trent

Woollett, Dosanjh-Matwala (1990) Postnatal care: the attitudes and experiences of Asian women in east London. *Midwifery* **6**: 178–84

Index

A

Abuse Assessment Screen (AAS) 107
Acheson, Donald 1, 3, 13
alcohol 7, 31
alcohol consumption 31
antenatal screening 42, 43, 44, 46, 48
assertiveness 6
assertiveness skills 24
asthma 9, 80
asylum seekers 21, 23, 28, 31, 32, 33,
        89, 91
  definition of 52
audit 22
Azaan 150

B

Baby Friendly Initiative 11
baby massage 24
Birth Companions 86, 87, 93
Black, Sir Douglas 3, 15
bottle-feeding 11
breastfeeding 4, 9, 10, 11, 12, 15, 18, 32,
        71, 87, 88
  as a public health challenge 10
breast screening 42

C

caesarean section 70
cancer 4, 8, 11, 13, 14
cervical cancer screening 42
children's centres 8

chorioamnionitis 103
clinical governance 153
communication
  problems for asylum seekers 61
community mothers schemes 4
continuity of care 54
coronary heart disease 4
cot death 7, 9
cultural awareness 103

D

dental checks 42
depression 53, 56, 57, 80, 101, 107
deprivation 3, 7
diet
  poor 5
disclosure
  of domestic abuse 111
dispersal 59
domestic abuse
  its impact on health 101
  its process 98
domestic abuse 95, 97, 98, 99, 100, 101,
        102, 105, 106, 111, 112, 113
domestic violence 7, 18, 21, 23, 24, 25,
        29, 30, 31, 36, 54, 55, 95, 96, 97,
        99, 101, 102, 103, 104, 105, 106,
        107, 108, 109, 110, 111, 112, 113,
        114, 115, 116, 117, 146
  definition 95
  detecting 106
  health professionals response to 104
  in pregnancy 102
drug abusers 18
drug users 90